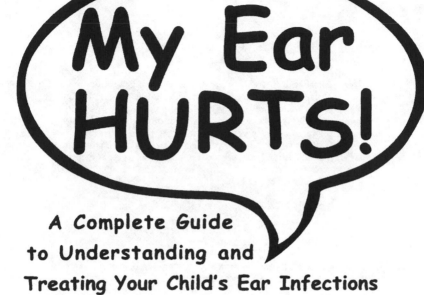

# My Ear HURTS!

A Complete Guide
to Understanding and
Treating Your Child's Ear Infections

Ellen M. Friedman, M.D., F.A.A.P., F.A.C.S.
James P. Barassi, D.C., D.A.C.B.S.P.

Illustrated by Patricia Shea

A CMD Publishing Book

A FIRESIDE BOOK
Published by Simon & Schuster
New York   London   Toronto   Sydney   Singapore

FIRESIDE
Rockefeller Center
1230 Avenue of the Americas
New York, NY 10020

FIRESIDE and colophon are registered trademarks
of Simon & Schuster, Inc.

For information about special discounts for bulk purchases,
please contact Simon & Schuster Special Sales:
1-800-456-6798 or business@simonandschuster.com

Designed by Christine Weathersbee

Manufactured in the United States of America

1   3   5   7   9   10   8   6   4   2

Library of Congress Cataloging-in-Publication Data

Friedman, Ellen M.
My ear hurts! : a complete guide to understanding and treating your child's
ear infections
/ Ellen M. Friedman, James P. Barassi ; illustrated by Patricia Shea.
p. cm.
Includes bibliographical references and index.
1. Otitis media in children—Popular works. 2. Children—Diseases—
Treatment—Popular works. I. Barassi, James P. II. Title.

RF225.F75 2001
618.92'09784—dc 21
2001034228

ISBN 0-684-87300-1

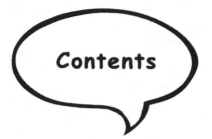

# Contents

Introduction 7

Chapter 1. What Is an Ear Infection? 9

Chapter 2. Causes and Risk Factors 32

Chapter 3. Taking Your Child to the Doctor 57

Chapter 4. Conventional Treatments: Medications 80

Chapter 5. Conventional Treatments: Surgery 105

Chapter 6. Complementary and Alternative Treatments 132

Chapter 7. Your Treatment Plan 160

Chapter 8. Preventing Ear Infections 183

Chapter 9. Parenting the Child with Ear Infections 215

Final Words of Encouragement 226

Resources 227

Index 233

## Introduction

"My ear hurts!"—is an all-too-familiar cry to many parents, who can recount stories of their young children waking up in the middle of the night with pain in their ear. This occurrence sometimes starts a chain of events that can leave both parent and child exhausted: sleepless nights, trips to the doctor, courses of antibiotics, repeat infections, discussions of other possible treatments. As a parent, it can be a frustrating experience if you do not understand all of the medical information presented by the pediatrician or do not feel comfortable with the suggested treatment. And in the case of ear infections, there are many conflicting reports as to what is the best treatment for this condition.

Conventional treatments often involve use of antibiotics or, in more severe or persistent cases, surgery. However, recent research suggests that some ear infections may be caused by viruses or allergies and not by bacteria, so antibiotics are not necessarily the appropriate treatment since they are only effective in fighting bacterial infections. The emergence of bacteria that do not respond to antibiotics—known as *antibiotic-resistant bacteria*—has also prompted calls for more selective and judicious use of antibiotics.

There has been a surge of interest in alternative treatments for ear infections—for instance, herbal remedies, homeopathic medicines, and chiropractic methods of spinal manipulation and massage. But for parents, choosing an alternative treatment can be a difficult decision. These treatments are still under debate in the medical community. Parents often turn to these methods without having full information about their effectiveness and in what cases their use may be appropriate.

Clearly there is no single right answer for how to handle an infection of the ear—every child is unique and every case is unique. The key is to select the best remedy based on the specifics of *your child's* particular case. One way to do this is to become more informed about some of the facts—and myths—related to ear infections: What causes ear infections? Why do some children have recurring ear infections? What are all of the treatment options—both conventional and alternative? How can you help prevent repeat ear infections in your child?

Equally important and challenging is to find ways to work in partnership with your child's doctor and other health care providers—asking questions, sharing knowledge of your child, and giving your input on decisions about treatment. By being an informed consumer and advocate for your child, you can make a valuable contribution to your child's health care.

While all of this will not ensure a childhood free of disease, it may start you on the road to feeling more informed and empowered in obtaining good health care for your children, and that will go a long way toward promoting their development and optimum good health.

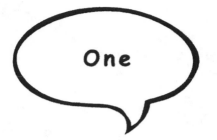

# What Is an Ear Infection?

## Anatomy of the Ear and Related Structures

In order to understand what happens when an ear gets infected, it is helpful to have a basic idea of the structure and function of the ear. This complex and delicate organ is composed of the outer ear, middle ear, and inner ear. The outer and middle ears function to conduct sound waves through the ear. The inner ear receives these auditory waves, transforms them into electrical signals, and relays them to the brain. The inner ear is also an important organ of equilibrium, or balance (see Figure 1).

### Outer Ear

The outer ear consists of the visible projecting flap of tissue and cartilage called the auricle or pinna, and the ear canal (external auditory meatus). The outer ear canal leads to a thin, translucent membrane—the eardrum (tympanic membrane), which senses vibrations created by sound.

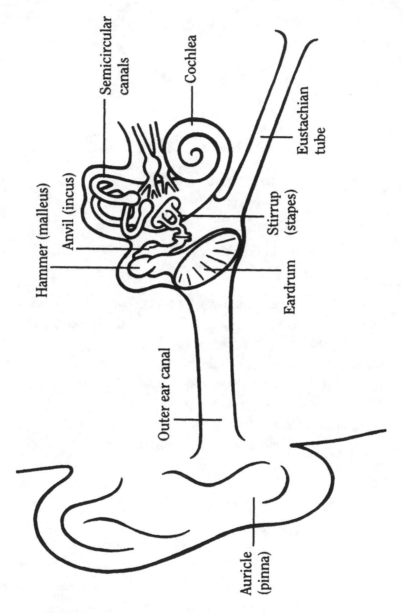

FIGURE ONE  Anatomy of the ear

## Middle Ear

Behind the eardrum is the middle ear, an air-filled cavity that contains a bridge of three tiny bones (ossicles) with the whimsical names anvil (malleus), hammer (incus), and stirrup (stapes). These bones—which are the smallest in the human body—are covered with a glistening membrane that constantly produces mucus. As the eardrum vibrates it moves the three bones, which then transmit the vibrations to nerves in the inner ear through a second thin membrane covering an area called the oval window.

## Inner Ear

The inner ear (labyrinth) is a coil or snaillike chamber with three sections. The central and upper sections of the inner ear contain the body's balance mechanisms (the semicircular canals). The lower section is a bony, snail-shaped structure called the cochlea. The cochlea has three compartments filled with special auditory liquids (perilymph and endolymph) that transmit vibrations received from the middle ear. The middle and smallest of these compartments contains the tiny auditory receptor called the organ of Corti. In this organ, tiny receptor cells (called hair cells) receive vibrations from the auditory liquids and relay the sound waves to auditory nerve fibers, which extend from the inner ear to the hearing center of the brain. These fibers transform the sound waves to electrical signals that are received and interpreted ("heard") by the brain. In this fascinating process, the brain can eventually distinguish over 400,000 sounds.

## Eustachian Tube

An additional structure that affects the middle ear—and plays a major role in ear infections—is the passageway that connects the middle ear to the nasal cavity and the throat. This passageway, called the eustachian tube, is more rigid closer to the ear and more pliant toward the back of the throat. The flexible end is normally closed at rest but opens very briefly upon swallowing or yawning. When the tube opens, air enters the canal and travels to the middle ear. The eustachian tube has three roles in regard to the middle ear:

> 1. **Ventilation:** The tube allows extra air to enter or leave the middle ear in order to keep the air pressure inside the ear roughly equivalent to the air pressure in the external canal. This function is most apparent when there are sudden changes in the outside air pressure, such as during travel through an underground tunnel or when taking off or landing in an airplane. If there were no such valve, rapid changes in middle ear pressure could cause the eardrum to rupture.

> 2. **Drainage:** The tube prevents buildup of normal mucus secretions in the middle ear by opening periodically to allow the excess fluid to drain to the back of the throat.

> 3. **Protection:** The tube provides partial protection from foreign substances that may be blown into the nose or throat region during

sniffing, sneezing, or coughing; when the tube
is closed at rest, it provides this protection.

Proper functioning of the eustachian tube helps to prevent damage to the eardrum and the middle and inner ears.
Inefficient functioning can lead to ear infection.

## Adenoids and Tonsils

Adenoids and tonsils are part of the body's lymphatic
system, a network of vessels, nodes, tissue, and glands that
plays a large role in defending the body against infectious
agents. Lymph, a clear, watery fluid derived from blood, flows
through this system. Special lymph cells (lymphocytes) that
originate in masses of lymph tissue (lymph nodes) protect the
body from infection by producing antibodies or by engulfing
and destroying foreign matter. Lymph nodes are concentrated in the throat, neck, chest region, armpits, and groin.
The tonsils are masses of lymphatic tissue located in the
throat near the back of the mouth. The adenoids are masses
of lymphatic tissue farther up the throat near the back of the
nasal cavity and cannot be seen through the mouth because
they are hidden behind the soft palate (the rear, fleshy part of
the roof of the mouth). During childhood the tonsils and adenoids work overtime, fighting off infections in the mouth,
nose, and throat regions. As a result, they can become infected
and swollen. The infection may travel to the middle ear. The
adenoids can also swell up and block the eustachian tube (see
Chapter 2). Moreover, when the tonsils or adenoids work
overtime and become larger, they may work less and less
effectively and become totally useless in the fight against
infections.

# Why Children Are Prone to Ear Infection

## Structure of the Eustachian Tube

One main reason why children are more vulnerable than adults to infections in the ear has to do with the structure and functioning of their eustachian tubes (see Figure 2).

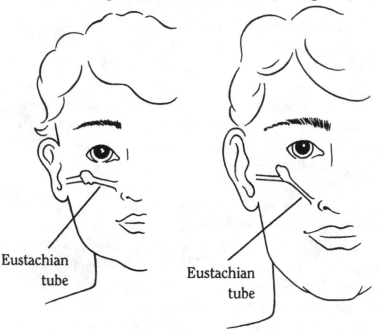

Eustachian tube

Eustachian tube

FIGURE TWO One reason that young children are more susceptible to ear infections is that their eustachian tubes are shorter and straighter and have a horizontal placement compared with the tubes of adults. This allows foreign substances to reach the middle ear more easily and makes it more difficult for mucus to drain from the middle ear. As a child grows, the tube becomes longer and angles downward, creating a more difficult path for foreign substances to reach the middle ear and allowing for easier drainage.

In adults, the tube is longer and slightly bent; the cartilage is more rigid, and the tube is angled downward at about 45 degrees from the middle ear to the throat. The length and bent path makes it more difficult for bacteria to reach the middle ear; the rigidity means less chance for swelling and blockages, and the downward angle allows for easier drainage of fluid down to the throat, all of which help to prevent infection.

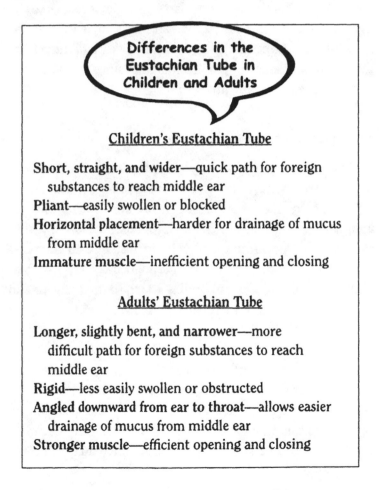

**Differences in the Eustachian Tube in Children and Adults**

### Children's Eustachian Tube

Short, straight, and wider—quick path for foreign substances to reach middle ear
Pliant—easily swollen or blocked
Horizontal placement—harder for drainage of mucus from middle ear
Immature muscle—inefficient opening and closing

### Adults' Eustachian Tube

Longer, slightly bent, and narrower—more difficult path for foreign substances to reach middle ear
Rigid—less easily swollen or obstructed
Angled downward from ear to throat—allows easier drainage of mucus from middle ear
Stronger muscle—efficient opening and closing

In young children, the tube is shorter and straight, making it easier for microorganisms from the mouth and nose to reach the middle ear. Since the tube lies at a nearly horizontal position, it is more difficult for accumulated mucus in the middle ear to drain into the throat. It is also easier for the immature tube to become obstructed or swollen because the tube is more pliant and the tiny muscle that ordinarily opens the eustachian tube also works less efficiently in infants. Adenoids are also more likely to block the eustachian tube in children. However, as a child grows older the eustachian tube's angle will become more vertical, its cartilage will become stiffer, and the muscle that controls the opening of the tube becomes stronger, thus eliminating much of the problem.

## Immature Immune System

Another major reason why ear infections afflict children much more than adults relates to the immune systems of infants and young children. Infants are born with numerous antibodies from their mothers. (Antibodies are protein substances made by white blood cells in response to the presence of foreign substances, *antigens,* in the body—such as viruses or bacteria. The antibodies attach to the antigens and destroy them.) These maternally "inherited" antibodies are present for about the first six months, helping to protect infants from infection, but they gradually diminish. By six months children start producing their own antibodies, but production does not reach a significant protective level until between the ages of one and two. This leaves a window between six and twenty-four months when children are most susceptible to bacterial and viral infections (such as colds), which can lead to ear infections.

Breast-feeding greatly helps to protect children during this vulnerable window. Breast milk contains special antibodies (immunoglobulins) that specifically fight infectious agents in the ears, nose, mouth, and throat. (The protective effects of breast-feeding are discussed further in Chapter 8.)

## Symptoms of Ear Infection

There are different kinds of ear infections and the symptoms vary accordingly. So in explaining symptoms, it is important to first clarify the distinction between these different infections. Infections can occur in the outer ear, the middle ear, and—rarely in children—the inner ear.

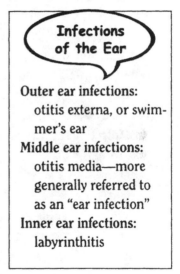

Infections of the Ear

Outer ear infections: otitis externa, or swimmer's ear
Middle ear infections: otitis media—more generally referred to as an "ear infection"
Inner ear infections: labyrinthitis

### Outer Ear Infection— Otitis Externa, or Swimmer's Ear

Infection in the outer ear is called otitis externa, which means inflammation of the external ear canal. Its common term is swimmer's ear. In this case, bacteria that normally live on the surface of the skin get beneath the skin and infect the outer ear. Bacteria can get through the skin barrier if the skin is scratched, cracked from dryness, or softened through prolonged exposure to water. As a result, the skin in the ear canal can become inflamed, itchy, or filled with pus, and usually drains purulent debris, which may have a foul odor. This is a common condition among children who swim often, and it can be treated by a doctor—usually by cleaning the ear canal and applying ear drops. The doctor may also prescribe earplugs and ear drops to be used when swimming to avoid future infections.

## Middle Ear Infection—Otitis Media

The general term *ear infection* usually refers to inflammation of the middle ear. The medical term for this is otitis media. In this condition any number of things—respiratory infections, irritants, allergies—can inflame the lining of the eustachian tube, producing swelling and increased secretions. When the tube becomes swollen or blocked it cannot function properly in draining the middle ear. Fluid can build up in the middle ear cavity, putting pressure on the eardrum, in some cases causing it to rupture. The accumulated fluid may be noninfected (sterile) or become infected and full of pus. Infectious agents can travel to the middle ear from the nose and throat via the eustachian tube or from the external ear canal through a hole in the eardrum, or perforated eardrum.

Otitis media can be grouped into two main types, each of which has an acute and chronic form. Acute refers to a sudden onset of symptoms, while chronic refers to a long-term condition. There can be variations within these types depending on what has caused the condition and how a child's immune system responds to it.

### Acute Suppurative Otitis Media (AOM)

In cases of AOM, the fluid that accumulates in the middle ear is infected by a virus or bacteria and can cause pus formation (suppuration). AOM often follows the common cold or other respiratory infections. Fluid can build up in one or both ears, often pressing strongly on the eardrum, and there is usually a rapid onset of one or more of the following symptoms:

- Ear pain, often severe and throbbing

- Fever

- Drainage or discharge from the ear

- Red or bulging eardrum

- Sleeplessness

- Irritability

- Lethargy

- Loss of appetite

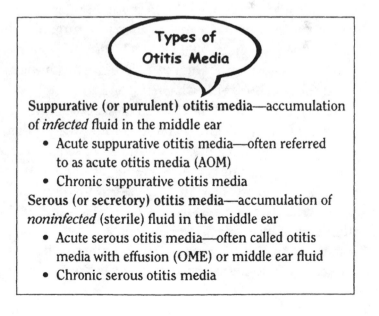

**Types of Otitis Media**

Suppurative (or purulent) otitis media—accumulation of *infected* fluid in the middle ear
- Acute suppurative otitis media—often referred to as acute otitis media (AOM)
- Chronic suppurative otitis media

Serous (or secretory) otitis media—accumulation of *noninfected* (sterile) fluid in the middle ear
- Acute serous otitis media—often called otitis media with effusion (OME) or middle ear fluid
- Chronic serous otitis media

However, AOM can behave very differently depending upon what type of bacteria or virus has caused the infection. Some are more aggressive than others. An invasion of bacteria coupled with one or more viruses can complicate the situation even more. (The differences between viral and bacterial infections are discussed in Chapter 2.) In addition, every child has unique symptoms, and parents may need time and intuition to interpret the signs correctly. For example, in infants, parents might notice slight redness in the ear. A young child might tug on an ear to indicate ear pain, but in another child this might just indicate anxiety or teething. One way to help distinguish general irritability from severe ear pain is that ear pain is usually more constant; a child may be hard to console, may rarely seem contented or playful, and may have great difficulty sleeping at night. If these symptoms persist for more than twenty-four hours, parents should take their child to see a doctor.

AOM is very treatable with antibiotics—when the infection is bacterial—or decongestants and mild pain relievers. If the ear pain is severe, a myringotomy—a surgical technique to drain out the middle ear fluid—may be performed to relieve pressure on a bulging eardrum. (Treatment for AOM is discussed further in Chapters 4 and 5.)

In some cases of AOM the fluid buildup inside the middle ear space becomes too great, and it ruptures the eardrum, leaving a small hole, or perforation. While this sounds rather alarming, especially for parents of young children, it is not usually a serious problem. In most cases, the infection is easy to clear and the perforation will usually heal itself within a week after the infection is gone. If the eardrum has burst, the ear pain will usually resolve, but there will be visible discharge from the ear canal.

### Chronic Suppurative Otitis Media

Chronic suppurative otitis media is less common in children; it most commonly occurs in adults who had ear disease in early childhood. Chronic suppurative otitis media usually results from untreated or recurrent AOM, and a perforated eardrum that fails to heal. Over time, bacteria from the external ear canal can enter the middle ear through the hole in the eardrum and keep reinfecting it. The main symptoms are a persistent discharge of pus from the ear—either odorless or with a pungent smell—and fluctuating hearing loss (signs of hearing loss are discussed later in this chapter under Complications).

Parents of children with recurrent or chronic AOM should watch for these symptoms and seek medical attention if they suspect chronic infection. Prompt treatment can avert potential damage to the bones in the middle ear, prevent long-term hearing problems, and reduce the risk of other possible complications. Oral antibiotics may not be effective because there are over twenty types of bacteria that may cause this infection—different from those that generally cause AOM—and many of these bacteria do not respond as well to oral antibiotics.

### Acute Serous Otitis Media—Otitis Media with Effusion (OME) or Middle Ear Fluid

Buildup of sterile fluid in the middle ear can occur if the eustachian tube is obstructed or if an episode of AOM does not completely resolve; one month after AOM, 40 percent of children still have middle ear fluid. OME may also accompany the onset of allergies. Depending on the individual child, the fluid may be thin and watery (serous), or it may be thick and mucuslike (mucoid). Researchers have not yet found any precise reason why some ears tend to produce thicker effusions, but this type of OME is known as "glue ear." This type of ear infection is usually referred to as "fluid in the ears" in distinction from an acute ear infection, or AOM.

Because the fluid is sterile there are generally no accompanying signs of fever or ear pain. In fact, many children with OME may not show any symptoms at all and often act as if they feel well. Only a few accompanying signs may be present:

- Plugged feeling in the ear

- Popping sensation when swallowing

- Fluctuating hearing loss or muffled sounds

- Possible speech problems

- Problems paying attention

Obviously, infants cannot describe these sensations, and even children of speaking age may not express them. So parents should not be surprised or feel that they have been neglectful if OME is diagnosed during a well-baby visit, as often happens.

The fluid may drain on its own in a matter of weeks or may require medical attention if it has not drained within a three-month period. Treatment may include draining the fluid through an incision in the eardrum—myringotomy (discussed in Chapter 5)—or possibly use of a decongestant if the OME accompanies allergies.

### Chronic Serous Otitis Media

Chronic serous otitis media or OME can occur if there is inadequate treatment of AOM. It can also occur when there has not been AOM, but when there are chronically enlarged adenoids, severe nasal allergies, or chronic sinus infections. There are usually no symptoms except for temporary hearing loss, which may be difficult for a parent to detect in infants or young children. Early treatment and consistent follow-up monitoring are recommended to avoid potential temporary or long-term hearing loss. Treatments may include myringotomies, removal of the adenoids, or insertion of tubes through the eardrum to allow drainage of fluid. If there are any concerns about hearing or speech development, even young children can be referred for reliable and formal hearing testing.

### Inner Ear Infection—Labyrinthitis

Inner ear infection—labyrinthitis—is a rare complication of middle ear infection; see page 31 for a brief review.

# Complications of Ear Infections

## Hearing Loss

Potential permanent hearing loss is the issue of most concern for parents of children with recurrent ear infections. However, parents should be reassured that hearing loss due to an ear infection is usually only temporary; when accumulated fluid in the middle ear drains, hearing usually returns to normal. There are two different types of hearing loss: conductive hearing loss and sensorineural hearing loss (see also Chapter 3).

Conductive hearing loss means that sound is poorly conducted across the middle ear space. The more fluid there is in the ear, the less space there is for the eardrum to vibrate, and the more poorly the three ossicles function. This results in a muffling effect; children can still hear but softer sounds may be missed or will not be clear. Short words spoken rapidly may also not be heard. This type of hearing loss is the most common form due to fluid in the middle ear. Usually, the hearing loss is temporary and hearing levels return to normal when the excess fluid drains from the middle ear. In very rare cases, if the condition goes untreated, the bones of the middle ear may become damaged. This can result in long-term hearing problems, which may be corrected through intricate surgery to reconstruct or repair the bones.

The degree of loss depends primarily on the volume of fluid that has accumulated. The more fluid there is, the more muffling there will be. There does not appear to be any difference whether the fluid is thick or thin. Another important factor is whether there is fluid in one or both ears. Fluid in both ears would cause more impairment. There is still some debate about the effect of hearing loss in one ear in children (unilateral hearing loss). This type of hearing loss may lead to nonspecific learning problems in school, which may range from mild to severe. Some children seem to be able to hear well enough to function without too much difficulty, and some children with unilateral hearing loss may have trouble determining the direction of sound in a crowded room since both ears function together to help pinpoint the location of sounds.

Sensorineural (nerve) hearing loss affects the functioning of the auditory nerves or the cochlea, meaning that the transmission of electrical signals to the brain is impaired. This type of hearing loss rarely happens due to ear infections, but is possible if the fluid in the middle ear exerts pressure on the lower membrane of the cochlea—the round window. Sensorineural hearing loss is permanent.

The duration of hearing loss due to ear infections can vary from one day to several months and may be difficult for parents to detect. Children are often unaware that they have muffled hearing; they may become very content with only soft sounds and adjust to the altered hearing. However, with some children, especially if their hearing loss is moderate, parents might notice a change in the child's behavior.

For children with AOM or OME, the best precaution is to have a follow-up doctor's visit. If the fluid remains for more than three months, it is a good idea to schedule a hearing test to determine if any loss has occurred; testing can be done at any time after birth. This initial assessment can also serve as a starting point for comparison in the future if the condition persists. Most doctors also routinely screen infants for hearing problems at well-baby visits during the first two years. The earlier a hearing loss is detected, the easier it is to treat and decrease the chances of possible delays in speech and language development.

**Signs of Possible Hearing Loss**

- Turning up the volume on the television/radio
- Moving closer to the source of a sound
- Acting inattentive when being spoken to
- Ignoring spoken communications
- Additional signs (if a child has begun speaking):
- Asking people to repeat what they have said
- Lip reading
- Difficulty following directions
- Slight changes in speech
- Unclear speech

## Delays in Speech and Language Development

In studying the relationship between hearing loss and delays in speech and language, researchers have gained some understanding of what can interfere with normal language development.

In the same way that the brain needs to "see" an image or object once in order to be able to recognize it the next time it is seen, the brain also needs to "hear" a sound once in order to recognize it and decipher it the next time it is encountered. This means that if infants miss out on certain key language sounds during a period of temporary hearing loss in their first year of life, their brain may have difficulty deciphering these sounds when heard later on; or if hearing is muffled, children may not be able to distinguish some of the subtleties of speech and language, such as tone or inflection. Missing these distinctions can also affect how children perceive and learn language.

Some studies have found that children with recurrent ear infections in the first three years of life tend to score lower in tests of speech and language than other children their age who have not had repeat ear infections. However, parents should be aware that such findings have limitations. It is sometimes impossible to determine if a child might have done poorly due to reasons other than fluctuating hearing loss. And there is no current research to indicate whether children who test poorly in speech and language at a young age will continue to test poorly at a later age if the degree of hearing loss persists.

Overall, it is still difficult to predict precisely to what degree fluctuating hearing loss might affect speech, as children are individual in their development in general. The crucial time for learning a particular sound may come at very different times for different children. If the hearing loss occurs at a less crucial time, it might have little effect on speech and language development. Much also depends on the degree and duration of hearing loss. Although there has been a great deal of research in this area, the results have not been conclusive. Therefore, it is a good idea for parents with children who have had recurrent episodes of AOM or OME during their first year to monitor language development for possible speech delays. Some basic guidelines have been established to identify potential problems.

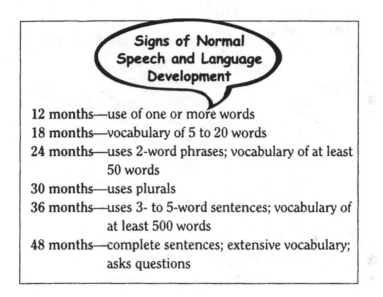

**Signs of Normal Speech and Language Development**

12 months—use of one or more words
18 months—vocabulary of 5 to 20 words
24 months—uses 2-word phrases; vocabulary of at least 50 words
30 months—uses plurals
36 months—uses 3- to 5-word sentences; vocabulary of at least 500 words
48 months—complete sentences; extensive vocabulary; asks questions

## Other Potential Developmental Delays

Some researchers have speculated that delays in speech and language development may also affect other aspects of normal child development, such as cognitive or social skills. This idea is based on the premise that speech and language problems can lead to poor communication skills, which may affect parent-child relationships, socialization with peers, and academic performance in later life. However, to date there is no conclusive evidence on whether—or to what extent—fluctuating hearing loss can affect such areas of overall development.

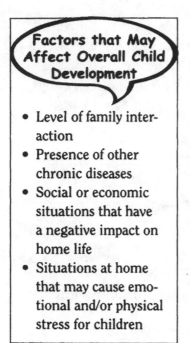

**Factors that May Affect Overall Child Development**

- Level of family interaction
- Presence of other chronic diseases
- Social or economic situations that have a negative impact on home life
- Situations at home that may cause emotional and/or physical stress for children

Parents should not assume that periods of temporary hearing loss necessarily mean long-term or irreversible problems in normal development for their children. The consequences of hearing loss can vary greatly depending on the individual child (see Factors that May Affect Overall Child Development).

In addition, there are numerous ways for parents to help counteract potential speech and developmental delays. With well-timed medical treatment and special attention to the child, most impairments can be overcome.

## Strategies to Counteract Potential Speech Delays

- Stimulate the child with stories, nursery rhymes, and singing.

- Encourage and reinforce speech.

- Address any situations or conditions that might be causing additional stress to the child.

- Involve the child in social activities, such as a play group.

- Make sure the child is receiving ongoing medical care to maintain good overall health.

## Mastoiditis, Meningitis, and Other Rare Complications

Other complications can develop if an acute or chronic ear infection spreads from the middle ear into the inner ear or other nearby structures. Two complications—mastoiditis and meningitis—are discussed briefly because of their potentially serious nature, but parents should keep in mind that serious illnesses occurring as a result of ear infections in the United States today are very uncommon.

### Mastoiditis

Mastoiditis occurs if an infection in the middle ear invades the mastoid process—part of the bone of the skull, located just behind the ear. The mastoid process has a network of air cells that connect to the middle ear space through a small opening in the back wall of the middle ear. A collection of pus may form, called an abscess, which may erode the thin, bony walls of the mastoid. The infection can then spread to other locations. If pus reaches the middle ear space it can be treated efficiently, but if the pus burrows under the skin or passes through to other bones of the skull, it can cause more serious infections.

Symptoms of mastoiditis are usually very apparent. Children generally have high fevers and the pinna (the outer ear)—or the skin behind the ear—may be swollen, red, or tender. The ear may also stick out, being pushed forward by the swelling over the mastoid. If parents suspect signs of mastoiditis, they should seek immediate medical attention; it needs to be treated aggressively with intravenous antibiotics and possibly surgery to remove the infected air cells.

*Meningitis*

Meningitis occurs when the protective tissue around the brain and spinal cord (the meninges) becomes infected. Microorganisms can invade the membranes lining the nose and throat and enter the bloodstream. Once there, they can travel to the blood vessels in the lining surrounding the brain. This infection can cause serious problems and requires immediate treatment.

Most children with AOM are not at risk of developing meningitis. However, as a precaution, parents should be aware of its early warning signs: persistent high fever, headache, nausea or vomiting, stiff neck, and lethargy (excessive sleepiness) or difficulty in being awoken from sleep.

If caught in the early stages, bacterial meningitis can be treated effectively with large doses of antibiotics administered several times a day over a period of ten days or more. Children in the United States now routinely receive a vaccination (called Hib—which refers to type b of the bacteria *Hemophilus influenzae*) that has significantly decreased the risk of meningitis caused by this organism. In addition, children as young as two months old can now receive a vaccine (Prevnar) effective against seven types of *Streptococcus pneumoniae*, a bacteria that is a common cause of both meningitis and ear infections. The use of these vaccinations may significantly decrease your child's risk for ear infections or complications from ear infections caused by these two common bacteria.

*Other Conditions*

Certain other conditions may result from repeated ear infections and persistent middle ear fluid. Chronic inflammation can cause scarring on the bones of the middle ear or on the eardrum (tympanosclerosis). Dead skin cells can build up behind the eardrum (cholesteatoma) and start to erode the ossicles. However, the majority of children do not experience such conditions; prompt treatment and follow-up after ear infections can prevent such occurrences.

Another rare complication of middle ear infection is labyrinthitis—infection of the inner ear; this can occur when an infection in the middle ear spreads into the inner ear, particularly into the semicircular canals. The main symptom is vertigo (a sensation of spinning in the absence of any movement); vomiting, nausea, and hearing loss can also be present. Parents who notice such symptoms should seek prompt medical attention.

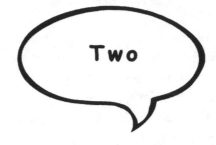

# Two

# Causes and Risk Factors

What causes an ear infection? It seems like a simple question, but the answer is not always so clear-cut. Infection occurs when the eustachian tube is not functioning properly or is blocked; fluid accumulates in the middle ear cavity, and foreign substances infect the fluid. However, a host of different factors may contribute to a dysfunctional eustachian tube and the resultant infection:

- Bacterial infections

- Viral infections

- Mechanical obstructions

- Allergies

- Nutritional deficiencies

The role of each of these contributing factors may vary with each infection. For example:

- Bacterial infections can come before or after viral infections.

- Viral infections may interact with nasal allergies to increase the severity or duration of the infection.

- Nutritional deficiencies may increase children's susceptibility to infections.

Moreover, remember that there are two types of middle ear infections. Buildup of infected fluid or pus in the middle ear (acute suppurative otitis media or AOM) is the most common form of ear infection that brings children to the doctor. The majority of cases of AOM are attributed to bacterial and viral infections. The second type of ear infection is characterized by accumulation of clear, noninfected fluid in the ear, known as serous otitis media or otitis media with effusion (OME). OME is thought to be caused primarily by incomplete resolution of AOM, obstruction of the eustachian tube, and allergic conditions.

As a result, each child's case is unique and it is sometimes difficult to identify the precise cause of a particular ear infection, which can be frustrating for both parents and doctors. However, working together, using some detective work—and sometimes a little bit of educated guesswork—parents and health care providers may be able to arrive at a more complete answer. Identifying the potential cause or causes of infection is just one of the many ways parents can help make informed decisions about what type of treatment is most appropriate for their child's particular case.

# Bacterial Infections

Bacteria are microorganisms that seek warm, moist climates to feed and multiply. They are present everywhere—in soil, water, plants, animals, and the human body. While bacteria are often thought of only as "germs," some bacteria have a beneficial function in the body. For example, bacteria present in the intestines help the body to digest food and eliminate wastes. It is only under certain conditions that bacteria infect the body, either internally or externally, and cause illness.

Infecting bacteria can enter the body through the nose and throat and reach the middle ear through the eustachian tube. When the tube opens and closes well and is not blocked, fluid drains into the back of the throat and is swallowed. However, during an ear infection, fluid builds up in the middle ear and bacteria become trapped and begin to increase rapidly. Even after the ear infection is treated, bacteria can still linger in the residual middle ear fluid for several weeks or months.

It is estimated that 70 percent of cases of AOM are caused by bacterial infection, either alone or with a viral infection. Analysis of the middle ear fluid in children with AOM has revealed that three main species of bacteria are responsible for the infection:

- *Streptococcus pneumoniae (S. pneumoniae),* an organism that is also associated with other diseases; it accounts for about 35 percent of cases of AOM.

- *Hemophilus influenzae (H. influenzae),* an organism commonly found in respiratory infections; it accounts for approximately 25 percent of cases of AOM.

- *Moraxella catarrhalis (M. catarrhalis),* a common inhabitant of the nasal cavity and throat; it accounts for roughly 10 to 15 percent of cases of AOM.

Antibiotics can be very effective in treating AOM. The type of bacteria that causes AOM is usually one of the three listed above, and an antibiotic effective against these species can be chosen. Vaccinating children as young as two months old against *S. pneumoniae* (to prevent the bacteria from causing an infection) is also now possible.

The bacteria that may be present in the ear of children with OME are slightly different. The three bacteria mentioned above are found in less than one third of the cases of OME. In other cases of OME, a wide variety of bacterial species have been found. Because it is harder to identify the infectious agent under these circumstances, antibiotics are not always considered an appropriate treatment, although there is still debate on the subject. Parents of children with recurrent OME may want to confer with their doctor about the possibility of allergic conditions or adenoid infections in their child; addressing these conditions could help to limit further episodes of OME.

# Viral Infections

Viruses are microorganisms that also cause infection, but unlike bacteria, they are not present in the human body most of the time and they are not killed by antibiotics. They also do not reproduce on their own; instead they enter the cells of a body and use their "host's" genetic material to multiply—sort of like tricking the cell into copying the virus instead of a new copy of a cell. In this way the virus multiplies and the cell is destroyed. Some of the most common viruses cause colds and the flu (influenza).

It is estimated that viruses alone account for at least 20 percent of cases of AOM. When viruses cause a cold or the flu, there are excess mucus secretions and inflamed membranes in the nose, throat, and eustachian tube. Mucus along with bacterial and viral particles may enter the tube, giving rise to infection and poor functioning of the tube. Mucus and inflammation may also block the tube, allowing buildup of fluid in the middle ear; viruses then multiply in this fluid. Secondary bacterial infections can also occur at this stage. However, identifying the particular virus is difficult. There are over 200 known common cold viruses and numerous variations (strains) of many of these viruses.

Treatment for a viral infection differs from treatment for a bacterial infection. Because of the unique way in which viruses multiply, antibiotics do not stop them. To date, vaccines have been the primary way to treat illnesses caused by viruses. In the United States, vaccinations have helped to virtually eliminate many childhood illnesses caused by viruses (for example, measles and polio). Creating vaccines to protect against the common cold and the flu has been difficult because of the enormous number of viruses involved. However, new antiviral drugs and vaccines are currently being tested and they may pave the way for more effective treatments of ear infections caused by viruses. (Vaccines are discussed further in Chapter 8.)

There is no easy way for the doctor to distinguish whether an ear infection is caused by a virus or bacteria, an important distinction because antibiotics do not work against viruses. Parents can discuss with their doctor whether antibiotics are suitable for their child's condition and also ways to relieve some of their child's symptoms. *Thoughtful use—but not overuse—of antibiotics is recommended for children with ear infections.*

## Mechanical Obstructions

Mechanical obstruction refers to blockage of the eustachian tube by swollen adenoids or tonsils. These clumps of lymphatic tissue work to support the body's immune system, producing lymphocytes, a type of white blood cell, which in turn produce antibodies to fight off infection. The tissues also trap substances from nearby areas that may be damaged from illness or from injury. Special white blood cells in the lymph nodes—called macrophages—fight infection by engulfing and destroying foreign substances. When bacteria, viruses, or other irritants enter the nose or throat areas, the tonsils and adenoids work overtime to fight the infection. As a result the tonsils or adenoids become swollen and tender, filled with collections of cells and their engulfed debris. The more illnesses or injuries a child has, the greater the chances of having enlarged (hypertrophied) adenoids. Often when the tonsils or adenoids become enlarged, they are less effective or totally ineffective in fighting infections.

In fact, when the adenoids enlarge, the eustachian tube may become physically blocked, because the adenoids are located in the throat near the opening of the tube. Blockage of the tube interferes with its ability to drain and ventilate the middle ear and is associated with cases of recurrent or chronic OME. Research on the effect of adenoidectomy (removal of the adenoids) suggests that the adenoids may contribute to eustachian tube dysfunction in two ways: due to enlargement leading to mechanical blockage and by acting as a reservoir for infection.

# Allergies

An allergen is a foreign substance (antigen) that causes a specific reaction or hypersensitivity in the body, which increases each time a person is exposed to the same substance. When allergens enter the body (either through the nose or through foods that are eaten), the body releases substances called histamines that cause dilation (widening) of blood vessels in the membranes of the nose and throat or on the skin. Typical symptoms of allergies are runny nose, watery or itchy eyes, sneezing, and wheezing; skin reactions can include patches of itchy skin or severe hives (itchy, raised red bumps). Many substances can cause an allergic reaction in children; some of the most common allergens are found in the home, outdoors, or in certain foods.

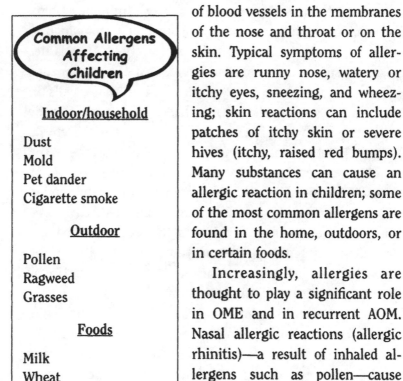

**Common Allergens Affecting Children**

**Indoor/household**

Dust
Mold
Pet dander
Cigarette smoke

**Outdoor**

Pollen
Ragweed
Grasses

**Foods**

Milk
Wheat
Nuts
Legumes

Increasingly, allergies are thought to play a significant role in OME and in recurrent AOM. Nasal allergic reactions (allergic rhinitis)—a result of inhaled allergens such as pollen—cause nasal inflammation, leading to eustachian tube dysfunction and increased secretion of mucus. In addition, there appears to be an interaction between nasal allergies and viral infections that enhances the process of infection. Moreover, some studies indicate that children with chronic OME often have some type of allergic condition. In several studies, a majority of children with recurrent OME were also found to be allergic to certain foods and when children stayed away from these items, there was significant improvement in their condition.

For parents with children who have recurrent OME, it is a good idea to consult with the doctor about the possibility of allergies as a cause or contributing factor; formal allergy testing is not recommended, however, for children under the age of three years. If subsequent testing of a child indicates allergic reactions to specific substances, treatment can include finding ways to eliminate or limit contact with those substances and, in selected children over age three, receiving allergy shots (immunotherapy). (See Chapter 8 for further information about treating allergies.)

## Nutritional Deficiencies

Although there is no conclusive evidence that nutritional deficiencies are a direct cause of ear infections, some findings suggest that certain minerals, vitamins, and fatty acids may play an important role in the proper functioning of the body's defense system against infections. Knowledge of the part nutrients play in health and in the immune system can provide parents with valuable information about their children's dietary needs. It is possible that by ensuring that their children have adequate quantities of needed nutrients in their normal diets, parents may be able to reduce the risk of ear infections.

## Mineral Deficiencies

Zinc is a trace mineral essential for the growth and repair
of tissue; a small amount is stored in the body, but there is
very little excess and it can be lost through sweating.
Findings suggest that zinc plays an important role in the
body's immune processes. The lymph cells (lymphocytes)—
which fight infection by producing antibodies—are activated
by zinc. Deficiencies in zinc can reduce antibody response
and cause weakening (atrophy) of the lymph glands. Zinc
deficiency has been found in children with frequent upper
respiratory and middle ear infections. Low zinc levels have
also been found in children with immunodeficiencies.

For parents who want to ensure that their children are
getting adequate zinc, fish, poultry, and meat offer concentrated doses that are easily absorbed by the body. For a meat-
less diet, the best sources of zinc are legumes, whole grains,
and milk products.

## Vitamin Deficiencies

There has long been speculation about the role of vitamin
deficiencies in connection with middle ear problems.
Vitamins A and E seem to have an indirect link. Vitamin A
helps maintain the lining of the upper respiratory tract; lack
of vitamin A can break down the cells of the membrane lining the middle ear and eustachian tube and can also destroy
the hairlike cilia that help move mucus and foreign substances out of the middle ear. Vitamin E plays an important
role in the functioning of the immune system and also helps
to regulate inflammation.

Parents can encourage their children to eat plenty of
squashes, melons, and green leafy vegetables—sometimes a

challenge for two- or three-year-olds with very definite tastes. All of these foods provide good sources of vitamin A. Vitamin E is found primarily in vegetable oils and nuts; wheat germ is also an excellent source of this vitamin. Infants are often given vitamin drops from age six months on; these generally contain generous amounts of vitamin A and E, and parents can feel reassured that infants are receiving adequate amounts of these vitamins. Parents should discuss with their doctor to what age vitamin supplements should be continued and whether it is necessary to provide supplements to older children, who can often receive adequate levels of vitamins through a well-balanced diet.

## Deficiencies in Essential Fatty Acids

Some fat in the diet is absolutely necessary to provide essential nutrients, known as essential fatty acids, that the body cannot manufacture itself. Essential fatty acids are needed for the body's growth and development. Omega-3 fatty acids, a particular type found in certain vegetable oils (especially canola oil, safflower oil, and walnut oil) and fish (especially salmon, herring, and mackerel), appear to play a role in both preventing heart disease and in the proper functioning of the body's anti-inflammatory system, which works to curb inflammation in the body, including in the linings of the nose, throat, and eustachian tube.

On the other hand, the consumption of trans fatty acid, a chemically altered fat found in many commercially prepared foods, usually in the form of "partially hydrogenated" oils and in margarine, may interfere with the body's anti-inflammatory mechanisms and also has been implicated in heart disease. Parents wishing to ensure a balanced intake of fatty acids in their children's diet and avoid excessive consumption of trans fatty acids can limit the amount of "fast" foods and commercially processed foods (such as doughnuts, crackers, and cookies) their children consume. In general, a well-rounded diet of healthy foods (discussed further in Chapter 8) will provide children with a good balance of needed nutrients; parents should speak to their doctor if they have any nutritional concerns related to fat consumption.

# Causes of Recurrence

Why do some children get so many more ear infections than others? This is perhaps one of the most frequently asked questions by parents, and the answer can be elusive. Numerous risk factors can make a child more vulnerable to repeat infection; these factors are discussed later in this chapter. Beyond such risk factors, four situations can set the stage for recurrent infection:

- Antibiotic-related issues

- Persistent residual fluid

- Chronic adenoid infection

- Partial immune deficiency

## Antibiotic-Related Issues

Both acute suppurative otitis media (AOM) and otitis media with effusion (OME) can recur or persist if the initial infection is not treated effectively. If antibiotics are used, there are four situations that can lead to an unresolved infection:

- The infection is not caused by bacteria.

- The antibiotic used was not effective against the type of bacteria causing the infection.

- The bacteria causing the infection has become resistant to the antibiotic.

- The antibiotic was not taken as directed—at the prescribed dose for the full length of time.

### Infection Not Caused by Bacteria

If the infection is caused *not* by bacteria but by a virus, allergen, or mechanical obstruction (or a combination of any of these three), then the antibiotic will not be effective; the infection will not resolve and the likelihood of recurrent infections rises. Allergies are most commonly associated with OME (sterile fluid in the middle ear) and not AOM.

### Antibiotic Not Effective Against the Type of Bacteria Causing the Infection

If an ear infection is caused by bacteria, antibiotics can kill most of the bacteria and speed up the body's natural healing processes. However, each antibiotic is effective against specific types of bacteria, and it can be a bit of a guessing game to determine which bacteria is causing the infection. Because the majority of AOM cases are caused by three bacteria (*S. pneumoniae, H. influenzae,* and *M. catarrhalis*), the doctor will start with an antibiotic that is known to be effective against these three; amoxicillin is a common first choice. But if the infection is caused by a different type of bacteria, amoxicillin may not work (see also Chapter 4).

### Bacteria Resistant to the Antibiotic

Even if the infection is caused by one of the three bacteria named above, amoxicillin or a similar antibiotic may fail to work, especially if it has been administered previously and the bacteria have become *resistant* to it. The emergence of such *antibiotic-resistant bacteria* is an area of great concern to health care providers and families alike. In order to understand how this happens, it is helpful to look at how bacteria and antibiotics function.

Bacteria are simple microorganisms whose main goal is to stay alive; they eat, they reproduce, and they fight off invaders. Bacteria have strong cell walls to protect them from attack and from any adverse conditions that may be present in the environment they are inhabiting. These cell walls contain special proteins that help bacteria to digest food and reproduce. Each cell contains genes (made up of DNA) that are used to duplicate new bacteria. Without these special proteins and genes, the bacteria could not multiply and spread infection.

Antibiotics inhibit or stop the growth of bacteria or fungi in one of three ways. They attack either the bacteria's cell walls, the special proteins, or the genes. However, bacteria learn quickly and can fight back with strategies of their own. If the bacteria have already encountered a specific antibiotic, over time certain strains of the bacteria may figure out ways to outsmart the antibiotic and stop it from working. These strains of bacteria are then considered "resistant" to this antibiotic. If this antibiotic is later used to treat an infection, the antibiotic will only be able to kill off strains of bacteria that are still sensitive to it; resistant strains of bacteria will thrive and multiply.

One of the main ways parents and doctors reduce the risks of children harboring antibiotic-resistant bacteria is by using antibiotics only when absolutely necessary. (Judicious use of antibiotics is discussed in Chapter 4.)

### Antibiotic Not Taken as Directed

Antibiotics may fail to work effectively if they are not taken as prescribed by the doctor—that is, at the full dosage for the full length of time. After a few days of taking the medication, a child may often feel better, and parents may decide to discontinue the antibiotic. But stopping the drug early may mean that the remaining bacteria are not killed, and this can lead to a recurrence of the infection. For the medication to work effectively, it is important that the treatment schedule be followed as prescribed. Parents need to talk to their doctor if any special situations occur (for example, a child refusing to take medicine or showing a reaction to the medicine, or if there is a difficulty in maintaining a three-times-a-day schedule) that may prevent the antibiotic from being given as directed.

## Persistent Residual Fluid

After an episode of AOM, if the fluid in the middle ear fails to drain completely and persists over a period of ten weeks or more, it is considered persistent residual fluid. The continuing presence of fluid in the middle ear creates an environment that leads to the multiplication of bacteria or viruses in the middle ear cavity, sets the child up for another infection, and causes a temporary hearing loss.

Residual fluid can linger in the middle ear for many weeks or months after the acute symptoms of an ear infection have passed: 20 percent of children still have some middle ear fluid present two months after an episode of AOM; 5 percent of children have residual fluid four months after an infection. Typically children do not experience pain or other symptoms with this condition, so parents may not be aware that there is a problem. If repeat ear infections develop in a child, follow-up visits with the doctor may be needed two months after the end of each infection to be sure there is no residual fluid. If fluid persists, treatments to drain the ears should be considered.

## Chronic Adenoid Infection

When air is breathed in through the nose, it comes through the nasal cavity and into the back of the throat, where the adenoids are located, then continues down the throat to the lungs. Adenoids are more prominent in children and generally decrease in size by puberty; few adults have adenoids. In children, these lymphatic tissues work to fight the numerous upper respiratory infections that are so common, especially during the winter season. Consequently, the adenoids are also constantly at risk of becoming infected themselves.

Infected adenoids can become enlarged and physically block the eustachian tube. Infected adenoids also harbor bacteria or viruses, and their close proximity to the opening of the eustachian tube provides an easy path for new infections to take hold in the middle ear. Infected adenoids can also obstruct the air passageways in

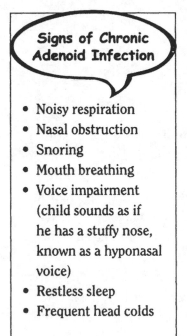

**Signs of Chronic Adenoid Infection**

- Noisy respiration
- Nasal obstruction
- Snoring
- Mouth breathing
- Voice impairment (child sounds as if he has a stuffy nose, known as a hyponasal voice)
- Restless sleep
- Frequent head colds

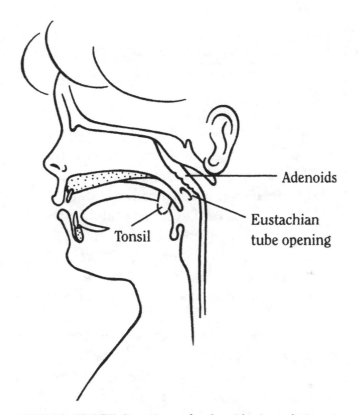

FIGURE THREE Location of adenoids in relation to eustachian tube opening. If the adenoids become enlarged, they can physically block the eustachian tubes. In addition, bacteria or viruses from infected adenoids can travel through the tube to the middle ear.

the throat and nose, resulting in chronic mouth breathing and snoring.

Parents of children with recurrent ear infections should be aware of some of the signs of chronic adenoid infection. If antibiotic treatments have not been effective at stopping recurrent infection, and there are signs of infected adenoids, the doctor may discuss the removal of the adenoids through a surgical procedure. (Adenoidectomy is discussed in Chapter 5.)

---

### A Personal Experience:
### Middle Ear Fluid

Steven and Michelle took their four-year-old, Kayla, to the doctor after a preschool hearing test revealed that she had reduced hearing in both ears. The parents had not noticed any signs of hearing loss and Kayla had been behaving normally.

The doctor carefully examined Kayla and explained to her parents that it appeared that fluid in her ears was the cause of her hearing loss. She reassured them that it was a condition that could be corrected and would not cause permanent loss of hearing.

Steven and Michelle were surprised that their daughter had middle ear fluid, since Kayla had never had any ear infections or problems with her ears before. A thorough history revealed that Kayla snored frequently and often breathed through her mouth. The pediatrician explained that Kayla's condition might be related to enlarged adenoids interfering with functioning of the eustachian tubes. He recommended that the next step was for Kayla to be examined by an otolaryngologist to evaluate the condition of her adenoids and by an audiologist for a more complete hearing assessment.

---

## Partial Immune Deficiency

The immune system provides the body's special defense response against foreign organisms. In addition to the network of lymph nodes and lymph vessels located throughout the body, this system includes two organs made of lymph tissue—the spleen and the thymus gland. The spleen is located next to the stomach in the upper left region of the abdomen. It stores blood, filters foreign material out of the blood, and activates cells that produce antibodies. The thymus gland is located in the chest region between the lungs. During fetal life and childhood it is quite large, but it becomes smaller with age. The thymus gland plays an important role in the body's ability to protect itself, especially during fetal life and the early years of growth. A poorly functioning thymus gland can impair a child's ability to produce the white blood cells and antibodies that fight against infection.

When foreign substances (such as bacteria) enter the body, a variety of special white blood cells act to fend off the infection by mounting a multilevel response formulated to attack the invading organisms. This response includes cells specifically made to ingest the invading organisms as well as other white cells made to produce specific antibodies to help combat the infection.

Most children develop antibodies when they acquire an upper respiratory infection—when they "catch a cold." But some children's immune systems are not as strong at resisting infection. If there are any disturbances in the function of the spleen, the thymus gland, or in the production of the white blood cells needed to fight infection, the body may not be able to produce the necessary defenses. Such conditions are uncommon, and may correct themselves in a few years as a child's immune system becomes more mature. If children seem to acquire illness very easily and very frequently, the doctor may refer parents to an immunologist (an immune system specialist).

# Risk Factors

A wide range of factors can increase the chances that a child will acquire an ear infection. These factors can be grouped into three broad categories—biologic factors, socioeconomic factors, and environmental factors. Becoming familiar with these potential "risk factors" may help parents, as they take steps to reduce the risks of repeated infections. Unfortunately, as vigilant as any parent can be, biologic factors cannot be changed.

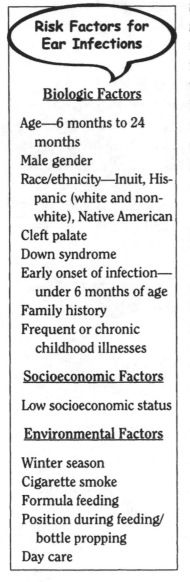

**Risk Factors for Ear Infections**

Biologic Factors

Age—6 months to 24 months
Male gender
Race/ethnicity—Inuit, Hispanic (white and non-white), Native American
Cleft palate
Down syndrome
Early onset of infection— under 6 months of age
Family history
Frequent or chronic childhood illnesses

Socioeconomic Factors

Low socioeconomic status

Environmental Factors

Winter season
Cigarette smoke
Formula feeding
Position during feeding/ bottle propping
Day care

## Biologic Factors

Even though parents cannot change biologic factors, all parents can take steps to minimize the potential risk for acquiring future infections by keeping up their children's overall health with regular checkups, vaccinations, prompt treatment of bacterial infections, and reducing or eliminating environmental risk factors.

*Age*

Children are most at risk for acquiring ear infections from six months to twenty-four months of age, due to the structure and function of their eustachian tube, and their immature immune systems.

### Gender

Studies have found that in general boys are more susceptible than girls to ear infections, although researchers have not yet identified the reasons for this difference. There are also exceptions; some families with several children report that their daughters have had more ear infections than their sons.

### Race/Ethnicity

Inuit, white and nonwhite Hispanic, and Native American children all have higher incidence of ear infections than other ethnic groups.

### Cleft Palate

In children with cleft palates (a condition in which the two bones that form the hard palate—the bony upper part of the mouth—do not come together normally before birth, creating a separation or split in the roof of the mouth), the tiny muscle that opens and closes the eustachian tube does not function efficiently. Therefore, the impaired eustachian tube will not be able to ventilate the middle ear space properly. The occurrence of OME in such children is almost universal. Parents of children with cleft palates or with any abnormality of the lip or palate should specifically ask their doctor to evaluate for middle ear problems. This will reduce the risk of potential hearing loss due to fluid accumulation.

### Down Syndrome

Nearly 60 percent of children with Down syndrome suffer middle ear problems. In children with Down syndrome, the muscle that controls the eustachian tube is impaired; poor eustachian tube functioning results in increased risk of ear infections.

### Early Onset of Infection—Under Six Months of Age

Researchers estimate that approximately 20 to 25 percent of children acquire an ear infection before they reach the age of six months. Some of these children are "high-risk" babies, meaning they were born prematurely or had low birth weight; some have associated bacterial infections and respiratory infections; a few have immunodeficiencies. Infection at such an early age can set the stage for a set of adverse conditions that greatly increase the risk for further infections. Immediately following the infection, the ear is more vulnerable to a new infection because

- There is fluid in the middle ear, providing a "good" environment for bacterial growth.

- The eustachian tube may be inflamed or blocked.

- The cilia (hairs) that help move mucus, bacteria, and viruses out of the middle ear may be damaged by the initial infection.

### Family History

Children with siblings or parents who have had recurrent ear infections in childhood have been found to have an increased risk of having repeat infections. Recent studies have found a strong genetic component to both the amount of time with middle ear fluid and the number of episodes of OME and AOM. This is most likely due to the way the face is shaped and the position and relationship of the eustachian tube to the throat and the middle ear.

*Frequent or Chronic Childhood Illness*

Children who contract upper respiratory infections are at greater risk for acquiring ear infections. In addition, if children have any chronic conditions, such as diabetes or a persistent cough, they may have an abnormality in their immune system, which may make them more vulnerable to other infections, including ear infections.

## Socioeconomic Factors

Social or economic situations that have a negative impact on children's living conditions can also pose risks for all kinds of illnesses, including ear infections. Crowded or unsanitary living quarters, poor nutrition, lack of access to medical care—situations such as these can have an adverse effect on the overall health of a child, making the child more susceptible to infection. A few large-scale studies have found higher incidence of ear infections among urban, lower-socioeconomic-status infants as compared with suburban, middle- and upper-socioeconomic-status infants. Incidence among children receiving Medicaid was also higher than among children whose families were enrolled in private health insurance plans.

## Environmental Factors

*Winter Season*

Ear infections tend to occur much more frequently during the winter months from December through March, largely because ear infections follow colds and other respiratory illnesses, which are more common during these months. It is felt that these illnesses are more common in the winter for several reasons. Cold air causes the blood vessels in the nose to swell, resulting in nasal congestion and eustachian tube dysfunction. Also during winter months, people are indoors much more frequently; the increased contact with other people in contained spaces makes the likelihood of passing and contracting viruses and bacteria much greater.

### Cigarette Smoke

Studies have shown that children who inhale secondhand cigarette smoke have an increased risk of ear infections. Secondhand cigarette smoke irritates the mucus membranes lining the nose, throat, and eustachian tube; exposure to smoke also damages the hairs (cilia) that are supposed to help move mucus out of the middle ear space; the result is a dysfunctional eustachian tube. In addition, cigarette smoke impairs the immune system by damaging the white blood cells that produce antibodies.

Some researchers have found a direct association between the number of smokers in a household and amount and duration of episodes of ear infections. Parents who smoke can reduce children's exposure to secondhand smoke by limiting their smoking to outdoor environments and keeping children away from public places where other people are smoking.

### Formula Feeding

Babies that are formula-fed rather than breast-fed have been found to have an increased risk of acquiring ear infections. Breast milk supplies babies with their mothers' antibodies; specifically immunoglobulin IgA, an antibody that attaches to the lining of the ears, nose, and throat and protects against many of the bacteria that cause ear infections. Breast milk also contains a protein called lactoferrin and enzymes called lysosomes that are effective at killing several types of bacteria. The cow's milk or soy protein used in most formula does not offer such protection. In addition, some children can get mild allergic reactions to formula; the resulting congestion and inflammation are conducive to the development of an ear infection.

When mothers are able to breastfeed their children, even for only three or four months, the protective benefits of breast milk may last even longer, supporting their child's growth and development. Mothers who are unable to breast-feed can find other ways to help protect their children, focusing on reducing other potential risk factors that may make their children more prone to ear infections.

### Position During Feeding/Bottle Propping

If children are given a bottle and allowed to feed while lying on their backs (sometimes referred to as "bottle prop-ping"), the fluid can be sucked up into the eustachian tube, carrying potentially dangerous bacteria to the middle ear. To avoid this problem, parents can hold their children at a more upright angle while bottle-feeding, keeping the child's head higher than the stomach. Parents should also make sure their children do not keep their bottles with them in their crib while napping or sleeping at night; in addition to its potential effect on the ears, falling asleep while bottle-feeding can also cause the milk to collect in the mouth and lead to the decay of emerging teeth (nursing-bottle syndrome).

### Day Care

Because children in day care centers are regularly in con-tact with many other children, they are more frequently exposed to infections than children cared for at home. Several studies have found a strong association between attendance at a day care facility and frequency of ear infections. Even children who do not attend day care, but whose siblings do, are at greater risk for ear infections.

For parents who use day care services, it is a good idea to try to choose a day care situation where the number of children does not exceed five or six; fewer children mean fewer risks of exposure to infection. Ask the care provider to notify parents if a child seems ill on a particular day so that the parent can come and retrieve their child, limiting the chances for the infection to spread. Some parents try to alternate care in a group setting with a baby-sitter who comes to the home. All of these strategies can help minimize the risks of frequent infection in day care.

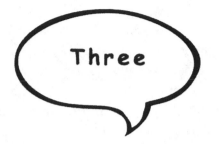

# Three

# Taking Your Child to the Doctor

## When to See the Doctor

As a parent, you may wonder when to call your doctor if you suspect signs of an ear infection in your child. You may not want to appear overanxious or make an unnecessary trip to the doctor if your child is not ill, but you also may be concerned about waiting too long and possibly neglecting an infection. While it can be difficult to find a good balance between these two options, there are a few general recommendations that can give you guidance in making decisions about when to see the doctor.

**Common Symptoms of Ear Infection**

- Ear pain
- Fever
- Drainage from ear
- Sleeplessness
- Irritability

If you notice signs of a possible ear infection (discussed in detail in Chapter 1), it is a good idea to wait at least twenty-four hours to see if the symptoms subside; 70 to 80 percent of untreated cases of ear infection self-resolve within twenty-four to seventy-two hours. Symptoms commonly occur during the night, so the twenty-four-hour rule can mean waiting at least through one more night to see if the symptoms persist—not an easy task for parents. If your child has ear pain or a fever, you can help her to feel more comfortable by elevating her head slightly, applying a warm washcloth to the ear (some children prefer a cool cloth, so you may have to test it both ways), and perhaps using a nonaspirin pain reliever, such as acetominophen or ibuprofen.

If your child's symptoms seem to be mild, you probably will be able to keep her comfortable and contented using some basic measures (also see Chapter 9). You may even be able to wait longer than twenty-four hours (but no more than seventy-two hours) to see whether the symptoms subside. You do not need to be worried that waiting a few days will make the infection more difficult to treat. In fact, studies have found that treatment by antibiotics is just as effective if it is delayed a few days. Waiting one to three days can also save you a needless trip to the doctor and possibly a course of antibiotics if the infection resolves on its own.

A few situations warrant more immediate medical attention. If your child's fever suddenly rises and stays high (above 102° F.), if her ear pain suddenly becomes severe and persists, or if you notice pus draining from the ear canal, it is important to call the doctor to notify him of the symptoms. If it is the middle of the night, the doctor may recommend some steps to alleviate your child's pain and have you bring her to the office in the morning. In general, it is not recommended to take your child to an emergency room in the middle of the night with ear pain. A potentially long wait in unfamiliar surroundings can increase your child's discomfort, and you also risk exposing her to other infections.

Decisions about when to see the doctor also reflect individual preferences of both parent and doctor. For example, a doctor may ask parents of a child who has already had several ear infections to contact him right away if they notice symptoms of a new infection. Some parents may prefer to call and check in with their doctor, even if they plan to wait one to three days before bringing their child in. Some doctors may also want to be notified if parents plan to give their child medication while waiting to see if the symptoms subside. You can discuss your preferences with your doctor when you first take your child in for a well-care visit before the actual situation arises; together you can arrive at an arrangement that suits everyone.

# What the Doctor Looks For

Going to see the doctor when your child has an ear infection can cause anxiety for both you and your child. Knowing in advance what the doctor's examination involves and how he makes his diagnosis may ease some of that anxiety. You can also help your child prepare for the visit by explaining a little bit about what will happen. Doctor's visits are covered in detail in Chapter 9.

## Otoscopy

The doctor's examination primarily consists of assessing how the eardrum looks and how it moves, through a procedure called otoscopy. The doctor uses an instrument called an otoscope to look into the ear canal and study the eardrum and middle ear. The doctor looks at a number of factors:

- Color of the eardrum

- Translucency of the eardrum

- Position of the eardrum—middle ear landmarks

- Movement of the eardrum

If there is a perforated eardrum, the doctor will make note of this during the exam.

### Color of the Eardrum

A healthy eardrum is normally a pale, shiny, gray color. Several types of changes in color can signal possible infection:

- Dull gray or blue indicates the presence of clear (serous) fluid in the middle ear.

- Yellow means mucus or pus is present.

- A "two-toned" appearance means the middle ear is only partially filled with fluid.

- Red may mean that there is an infection or a high fever or that the child has been crying vigorously.

While a red eardrum is considered a classic sign of acute suppurative otitis media (AOM), the color red does not *always* signal infection. Children can have a red eardrum due to crying, sneezing, or a fever. In fact, one of the most common reasons for an incorrect diagnosis of ear infections is that the diagnosis is made based on eardrum color alone.

### Translucency of the Eardrum

The eardrum is normally translucent like a frosted window but not totally transparent like a clear glass window. The doctor gauges translucency by checking whether or not he can see one of the three bones (ossicles) of the middle ear—the "short arm" of the hammer bone. When the eardrum is translucent, this landmark is easily visible and there is not likely to be any fluid in the middle ear; if this landmark cannot be seen clearly, there is probably an accumulation of fluid.

When the doctor looks through the eardrum into the middle ear, he may also see tiny air bubbles in the middle ear cavity, signaling the presence of fluid. Air bubbles can indicate impending resolution of the middle ear problem or otitis media with effusion (OME). An air-fluid level means that the middle ear space is only partially filled with fluid.

### Position of the Eardrum—Middle Ear Landmarks

The position of the eardrum gives the doctor an indication of how much—if any—fluid is present in the middle ear. Normally the eardrum is stretched flat across the opening to the middle ear; there is no fluid present and the short arm of the hammer bone is visible. However, if a little fluid has accumulated in the middle ear, the eardrum may begin to stretch outward slightly (away from the middle ear). The short arm of the hammer bone will not be visible; only the long arm can be seen. If the middle ear is completely filled with fluid, the eardrum may bulge severely outward and the doctor will not be able to see the middle ear landmark at all.

Sometimes, the eardrum is pulled slightly *into* the middle ear—called a concave or retracted eardrum; the short arm of the hammer bone will now look more prominent, and the long arm will appear small. A concave eardrum may denote a buildup of fluid or that the eustachian tube is blocked; air is not reaching the middle ear cavity, creating a vacuum effect that sucks the eardrum inward.

### Movement of the Eardrum—Pneumatic Otoscopy

In pneumatic otoscopy the doctor squeezes a little rubber bulb attached to the otoscope, blowing a tiny bit of air into the ear canal and sucking it out again; a normal eardrum should move slightly in and out with this action. If the eardrum does not vibrate normally, fluid is likely present in the middle ear; the less the eardrum moves, the greater the volume of fluid may be. Reduced eardrum vibrations can also signal a blocked eustachian tube; air is trapped in the middle ear, creating a sealed cavity, and the eardrum cannot move well.

### Perforation of the Eardrum

In a few instances, the doctor may see that the eardrum has already ruptured from excessive buildup of fluid in the middle ear. A hole of variable size is visible in the eardrum and most of the fluid will have drained out of the ear canal. (Perforation of the eardrum is discussed further in Chapter 1.)

## Additional Tests

If diagnosis through otoscopy and pneumatic otoscopy is inconclusive, the doctor may conduct additional tests.

### Tympanometry

Tympanometry assesses the functioning of the middle ear. A rubber plug is inserted into the ear canal and is attached to a machine called a tympanometer, which transmits sounds to the eardrum and middle ear and measures the amount of sound bounced back to the ear canal. This measurement is plotted as a curve on a graph, called a tympanogram. A normal eardrum will transmit vibrations to the middle ear; very little sound will be bounced back to the external canal. A fluid-filled middle ear will decrease the eardrum's transmission of sound waves and increase the amount of sound reflected back to the machine.

*Acoustic Reflectometry*

Acoustic reflectometry performs a similar function to tympanometry. A small handheld instrument (called an acoustic otoscope) is positioned at the ear canal. The acoustic otoscope emits a sound, which then bounces back to the machine; the characteristic of the reflected sound wave is displayed directly on the back of the instrument.

# Potential Difficulties in Examination

Conducting an ear examination on an infant or a very young child can be a challenge at times for both doctors and parents. Several factors can hinder examination:

- Child is moving or crying; in addition the parent may be concerned that the exam will physically or emotionally harm the child

- Shape and size of ear canal

- Differences in eardrums

- Wax in ear canal

Parents wishing to examine their children's ears at home with an otoscope should also be aware of these difficulties.

## Child Is Moving or Crying

If your child is moving around a lot, it may be difficult for the doctor to get a thorough view of the ear through the otoscope. Crying also causes the eardrum to turn red, making it

Home Otoscopes—
a Questionable Tool
for Parents

Some parents want to check their children's ears themselves with a home version of an otoscope. However, the type of home otoscope you can buy through a drugstore or medical supply store is of much poorer quality than the doctor's instrument: the amount of light generated is much less and the home otoscope can only check color and translucency (not mobility) of the eardrum. In addition, it is very difficult for a parent to know what to look for in the ear; even an experienced doctor may have difficulty interpreting what he sees through a good otoscope. For these reasons, home exam is not considered very useful and is generally not recommended.

If you wish to use a home otoscope, you should discuss it with your doctor first. Also keep in mind that a home exam is not accurate enough to use as an initial diagnosis, nor is it acceptable for follow-up monitoring. You still need a doctor to check your child's ears.

impossible to determine the actual color of the eardrum. During the examination, you can help by holding your child's head or letting her sit in your lap. Talking to and comforting your child can calm her and help minimize crying. Some parents are concerned that the exam may harm their child—either physically or emotionally—and they may interfere with the progress of the exam; ear examinations are safe procedures, however, and calmness on the part of the parent can help the child stay calmer also.

## Shape and Size of the Ear Canal

Ear canals come in a variety of shapes and sizes; tiny, narrow, or curvy ear canals make it more difficult for the doctor to get a good view of the eardrum and the middle ear. If the doctor is having trouble getting a proper look at your child's ear, stay relaxed, comfort your child, and allow the doctor to take his time. A little extra time is well worthwhile for accurate diagnosis and is far better than a rushed exam.

## Differences in Eardrums

Just as every child is unique, so is every eardrum, and there can be great variations in the appearance of normal— and infected—eardrums, depending on the child. It takes an experienced doctor, who has looked into hundreds of ears, to assess the condition of the eardrum accurately.

## Wax in the Ear Canal

If the ear canal is blocked with wax, impeding the doctor's view, he may try to flush it out with a special ear-cleansing syringe, with gentle suction, or by using a long thin instrument with a rounded tip, called a curette. Clearing wax can be time consuming and may add to your child's discomfort, so keeping your child calm and still during the procedure will help the cleaning go more smoothly.

If you want to help prevent buildup of wax in your child's ear on a regular basis, you can wipe the outer ear daily with a washcloth to remove the excess wax that comes out of the ear canal. However, you should never use a cotton-tipped swab to try to remove wax in the ear canal; such efforts only push wax farther into the canal, and there is a real risk of damaging the eardrum if your child moves suddenly. There are special drops available without a prescription that will also help to remove wax from your child's external canal; speak to your doctor if you are contemplating using drops to prevent wax buildup.

# Diagnosis

In spite of the possible difficulties in examining your child's ears, the doctor should be able to make a diagnosis after otoscopy, possibly with the addition of tympanometry. Remember that the two most common types of middle ear infections are acute suppurative otitis media (AOM), characterized by a buildup of *infected* fluid in the middle ear, and otitis media with effusion (OME), characterized by a buildup of *sterile*, uninfected, fluid in the middle ear. When the doctor gives his diagnosis, feel free to ask him questions about what he saw during his exam:

• Are there signs of fluid in one (or both) ears?

• Does the fluid seem infected or is it sterile (serous)?

• Is the eardrum in a normal position, or is it retracted or bulging?

• Is there a perforation of the eardrum?

Once the doctor has made his diagnosis, he will want to discuss treatment options with you. Feel free to ask questions and voice your preferences and concerns regarding suggested treatments. Clear communication fosters greater understanding between parents and doctors, and results in decisions about treatment that are acceptable and agreeable to both parties. You can also discuss preventive measures with the doctor to help reduce the chances of recurrent infection. (Prevention is discussed in Chapter 8.)

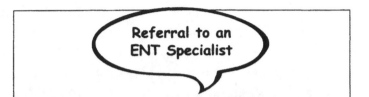

**Referral to an ENT Specialist**

If your child has had several repeat infections and has not responded well to antibiotic treatments in the past, your doctor may refer you to an "ear, nose, and throat" specialist (otolaryngologist or ENT doctor). The ENT doctor will confer with you and your primary care doctor about your child's medical history, particularly concerning ear, nose, and throat problems. In addition to conducting otoscopy and tympanometry, the ENT doctor will

- Examine the nasal cavity for signs of allergy or chronic infections
- Examine the mouth and throat for abnormalities in the lips or palate
- Assess speech and voice quality
- Examine the ears

The ENT doctor will try to pinpoint what is causing the recurrent infections and discuss with you appropriate strategies for prevention and treatment. If the ENT doctor or the primary doctor suspects possible hearing impairment, he may refer your child to an audiologist for hearing tests.

If your child has already had several ear infections, the doctor will want to know more about her medical history and her exposure to potential risk factors. Try to offer as much information as possible about previous illnesses, allergies, child care situations, environmental irritants (such as smoking), and any other factors that you think may be relevant to your child's case. Working with the doctor, you may be able to identify some underlying conditions (such as allergies) that need to be addressed or investigated further. In some cases, the doctor may refer you to an ear, nose, and throat specialist or, if extensive hearing testing is needed, to an audiologist (see page 71).

# Hearing Tests

### Ongoing Screening Tests

Screening to check that hearing is normal should be done by your baby's doctor at well-baby visits from birth onward; in some states newborn hearing screening tests are required by law. Speech and language progression should also be assessed during well checkups. Catching signs of hearing impairment at the earliest stages is the best way to prevent delays in language development and to decrease the severity of speech problems. For children over three to four years old, many preschools and grammar schools conduct regular screening programs to test hearing and vision. If any problems are noted, the school will recommend that your child see a doctor for further testing.

## Suspected Hearing Loss

Besides screening tests, other situations may indicate potential hearing loss and the need for a hearing test.

- **Persistent middle ear fluid:** If fluid in the middle ear remains longer than ten weeks after the end of an infection, there is the possibility that a child's hearing may be affected.
- **Behavioral problems:** A child may become frustrated, inattentive, or uncooperative if hearing problems are present.
- **Speech or language delays:** Changes in speech or signs of disruption in normal language development may signal hearing loss.
- **Parental concern:** Occasionally none of the above signs are obvious, but as a parent you may have an intuition that something is not right with your child. In these cases, it is a good idea to discuss the matter with your doctor. However, keep in mind that even a parent's intuition can be incorrect at times. Studies have shown that some parents may think their child's hearing is abnormal when it is actually normal; other parents think the hearing is normal, when it is actually abnormal. Only with reliable formal testing can one be sure.

## Preliminary Tests with the Doctor

If you suspect hearing loss in your child, call your doctor to discuss the matter and arrange for some preliminary testing, which will include:

- **Sound localization:** The doctor will shake a toy or

rattle outside your child's range of vision to see if she can detect where the sound is coming from; in-ability to locate a sound is an indicator that one (or both) ears may not be functioning properly. This test, however, is rather primitive and cannot be relied. upon as proof of normal hearing. If you are concerned about your child's hearing or have a positive family history for hearing problems, request an audiogram (see page 72).

- **Speech and language assessment:** The doctor will ask you a brief series of questions about your child's speech and language. Questions regarding infants could include the following: Is she quieted by a familiar voice? Does she respond to talking by looking at the person speaking? Does she make vocal sounds when played with? The doctor may note basic characteristics, such as the quality of your child's voice, her pronunciation, and her articulation of words. He may ask you about her vocabulary, her use of sentences, and whether she seems able to communicate effectively with other children her age. If the doctor detects abnormalities in speech, or if you have concerns about your child's language development, he will refer you to a speech language pathologist, a specialist trained to identify and treat speech and language problems.

- **Tympanometry:** The doctor may use a device called a tympanometer (see page 75) to assess the movement of the eardrum and to test middle ear function. This basic assessment, however, does not provide direct information about hearing; instead it shows whether or not there is fluid in the middle ear, which does not give specific information concerning hearing.

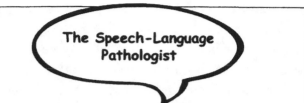

The Speech-Language Pathologist

A speech-language pathologist is a specialist trained to identify specific problem areas in your child's speech and language and to determine the appropriate therapies to address the problems. The therapist will test your child for pronunciation of words, use of language, language comprehension, and how she expresses herself. The therapist will also assess your child's voice quality and the rate at which she speaks. In addition, she will evaluate your child's social and emotional behavior by playing with your child and watching her interact with you. After evaluation, the therapist will design and implement a treatment plan to improve your child's speech and use of language.

When you receive referrals for a speech-language pathologist (from the audiologist or your child's doctor), try to select a therapist who specializes in working with children. The therapist should also be certified by the American Speech and Hearing Association and should be licensed by the state in which she works.

## Hearing Tests with an Audiologist

If you or your doctor is concerned about hearing impairment in your child, he will refer you to an audiologist—a specialist trained to evaluate the degree and type of hearing loss. Whenever possible you should get a referral for an audiologist who specializes in children's hearing disorders, or who at least has some experience working with children.

A hearing test will be scheduled with the audiologist *after* your child's infection is over; hearing tests are not conducted during an acute infection. On the day of testing, the audiologist will talk briefly with you and your child before starting the testing and explain a little about the tests to be conducted. He will take you and your child to a soundproof room; he may be in the same room or an adjacent room. During the tests, he will sometimes put earphones on your child; earphones are necessary to assess the hearing function in *each* ear separately, as opposed to the combined hearing of both ears.

The audiologist may use several different methods to assess your child's hearing:

- Audiometry—testing responses to levels of tones and sounds

- Bone oscillator or otoacoustic emissions (OAE)— testing inner ear function

- Behavior observation

- Auditory evoked responses

The audiologist will also use tympanometry to test middle ear function.

### Audiometry

The audiologist will use a machine called an audiometer to measure the sharpness and range of your child's hearing; the results are recorded on a graph, called an audiogram. Audiometry can assess the threshold of a child's hearing (the quietest tone or speech that the child can hear). The audiometry tests are behavioral assessments of hearing, meaning that the child's response to hearing sounds is observed.

The audiologist may use a technique called visual reinforcement audiometry (VRA) with infants or children who do not yet talk. A toy or other object in the soundproof room will light up when the audiologist speaks—first through a set of external speakers in the room, and later through the earphones. By setting it up as a game in which the light and object accompanies a sound, the audiologist can gradually coax your child to look at the object when she hears a word or tone. The audiologist will gradually decrease the volume of sounds and note when your child no longer looks up at the object. If your child is crying or unresponsive during the test, you can try to comfort and calm her. Do not worry that the test is not working; the audiologist may still be able to notice a slight pause or difference in crying when your child actually hears a sound.

For children over three years old, the audiologist may use a variety of techniques. In conditioned play audiometry (CPA), children are asked to put an object in a box or move a block each time they hear a tone. The audiologist may also ask your child to raise her hand when she hears a sound or repeat words spoken to her until she can no longer hear them. The audiologist may use two, three, or more such behavioral methods to reduce the possibility of incorrect results, particularly in the case of a child who seems inattentive or uncooperative. You can help by encouraging your child to play along, or even playing with her the first few times, with the audiologist's permission.

### Bone Oscillator or Otoacoustic Emissions (OAE)

The audiologist may use one of two tests to assess your child's inner ear. A bone oscillator is similar to earphones except that it is placed *behind* the ear; the oscillator measures the range of sounds picked up by the inner ear (the cochlea). In otoacoustic emission (OAE) testing, a small earphone and microphone are placed in the ear canal; a normal inner ear should respond to sounds with an echo that is picked up by the microphone. Deviations in normal functioning of the inner ear may indicate sensorineural (nerve) hearing loss, but this type of hearing loss is not common in children whose only indication is an ear infection. (Sensorineural hearing loss is discussed in Chapter 1.)

### Behavior Observation

During the hearing tests, the audiologist will also make general observations about your child's behavior: how she responds to requests; how she interacts with you, how she acts with him (a stranger). After the tests, he may also ask you about behavioral issues: whether your child has seemed inattentive or uncooperative; whether a baby-sitter or teacher has noticed any changes in your child's behavior. While it may feel a little uncomfortable discussing possible behavioral problems, by sharing such information, you can help the audiologist with his assessment.

### Auditory Evoked Responses

In auditory evoked response testing (also called brainstem auditory evoked potentials, or BAER), the audiologist places small electrodes (sensors) on your child's scalp. The electrodes record brain wave activity in response to clicking sounds your child listens to through earphones. The procedure is safe and painless and can be used even on newborns. Results, seen as a graph, show how different parts of the brain's auditory pathways respond to sound and can be used to determine the site of any damage along the pathways. Auditory evoked response testing may involve sedation so that your child is quiet or sleeping during the procedure, as any kind of head or neck muscle movement can adversely affect the results.

### Tympanometry—Testing the Middle Ear

The audiologist will use a tympanometer to test the function of the middle ear. This testing, which does not provide direct information about hearing, is more extensive than the basic tympanometry used by the doctor during a routine ear examination. In addition to evaluating the movement of the eardrum, the audiologist will assess whether the eustachian tube is working properly and whether the acoustic reflex is working (the stirrup bone in the middle ear should contract in response to loud sounds).

## Evaluating Hearing Loss

By the end of the session with the audiologist, she should be able to tell you:

- Whether the hearing loss is conductive, sensorineural, or a combination of both (see Chapter 1)

- How the middle ear and eustachian tube are functioning

- Whether there are problems in one or both ears

- The degree of hearing loss

To get a better understanding of what hearing loss means, it is helpful to look at how sound is mea-

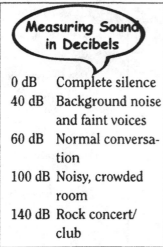

**Measuring Sound in Decibels**

| 0 dB | Complete silence |
| 40 dB | Background noise and faint voices |
| 60 dB | Normal conversation |
| 100 dB | Noisy, crowded room |
| 140 dB | Rock concert/ club |

sured. The intensity of a sound is measured in decibels (dB).

The degree of hearing loss is measured by the threshold level (the lowest tone a child can hear); the higher the thresh-

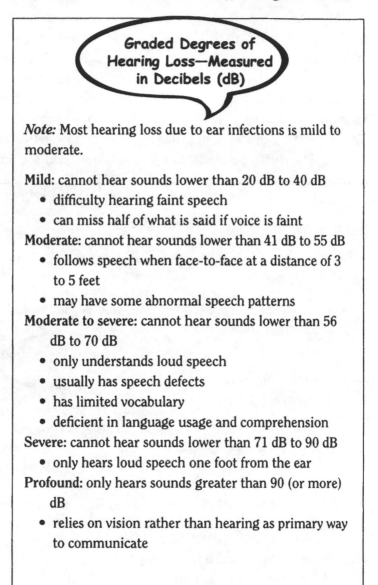

### Graded Degrees of Hearing Loss—Measured in Decibels (dB)

*Note:* Most hearing loss due to ear infections is mild to moderate.

**Mild:** cannot hear sounds lower than 20 dB to 40 dB
- difficulty hearing faint speech
- can miss half of what is said if voice is faint

**Moderate:** cannot hear sounds lower than 41 dB to 55 dB
- follows speech when face-to-face at a distance of 3 to 5 feet
- may have some abnormal speech patterns

**Moderate to severe:** cannot hear sounds lower than 56 dB to 70 dB
- only understands loud speech
- usually has speech defects
- has limited vocabulary
- deficient in language usage and comprehension

**Severe:** cannot hear sounds lower than 71 dB to 90 dB
- only hears loud speech one foot from the ear

**Profound:** only hears sounds greater than 90 (or more) dB
- relies on vision rather than hearing as primary way to communicate

old level is (measured in decibels), the higher the degree of hearing loss. As a frame of reference, normal background noise is about 40 dB and normal conversation is 60 dB. Conductive hearing loss due to ear infections is usually mild to moderate—a loss of between 15 to 40 dB. So if a child has a 25 dB loss, a normal conversation might sound more like background noise coming from another room.

Ear infections usually result in temporary hearing losses that are mild to moderate. Threshold levels are also measured at several frequencies (pitches)—noted in hertz (Hz). Hearing loss within specific frequency ranges can affect language comprehension. For example, the *s* sound is pitched at a frequency of 4,000 to 8,000 Hz. If your child's hearing is impaired in that frequency range, she will not hear *s* sounds properly. Inability to hear certain frequencies can also result in muffled or distorted hearing.

## Monitoring Hearing Loss

If your child is experiencing long-term or chronic ear infections, hearing tests should be conducted every three to six months to assess any changes in the degree or type of hearing loss. Periodic testing can also be used to evaluate the effectiveness of treatment. For example, if your child has tympanostomy tubes inserted (see Chapter 5), subsequent hearing tests can indicate whether your child's hearing has improved significantly since the surgery.

# Following Up with Your Doctor

After your child has had an ear infection, it is important to follow up with your doctor to make sure the treatment was effective and to catch any new infections that can occur following an initial ear infection. The correct time for a follow-up visit is controversial; however, it would be wise to see your doctor two to three months after AOM to be sure that there is no OME or fluid still in your child's ears. If you have already been referred to an ENT doctor, then follow-up could be with him, rather than with your primary care doctor.

## Follow-up for Cases of AOM

If your child was diagnosed with AOM and an antibiotic was prescribed, she should feel better within forty-eight to seventy-two hours of starting the course of medication. If your child is not feeling better after three days of medication, bring her to the doctor for a follow-up evaluation. Symptoms that persist usually mean that the antibiotic is not working, and the doctor will discuss with you further treatment options, such as use of a different antibiotic.

If your child is doing fine at the three-day point and appears to be responding to the antibiotic, you will not need to bring her to the doctor immediately. Instead, discuss with your doctor when to schedule a follow-up visit to see whether there is any residual fluid in the middle ear. Checking for fluid after six weeks is most useful because at that time additional testing or treatment may be needed.

If your child's symptoms resurface just a few days after the end of the course of antibiotics, you should notify your doctor. The original infection may not have resolved completely and the doctor may need to prescribe a different antibiotic. However, if symptoms appear more than a week after the end of antibiotic treatment, it is most likely a new ear infection and the doctor will need to reexamine the ear and make a new diagnosis.

## Follow-up for Cases of OME

If your child was diagnosed with OME, follow-up is different than for AOM. Remember that OME often occurs following an episode of AOM: 40 percent of children have fluid in the middle ear one month after an initial ear infection; 20 percent have fluid two months later; and 5 percent have fluid four months later. Discuss with your doctor when to schedule visits for OME follow-up.

If the doctor finds that fluid persists for longer than three months, he will refer your child for a hearing test with an audiologist to determine if the fluid is causing hearing problems. If hearing loss is mild—measured at a threshold level of less than 20 decibels—it means that the OME is not causing major problems in hearing. The doctor will continue monitoring your child every two months and refer you for periodic hearing tests to make sure that her hearing does not change for the worse.

If hearing loss is measured at 20 decibels or more, the doctor will discuss further treatment options with you, including use of antibiotics or surgery to insert tympanostomy tubes (see Chapter 5).

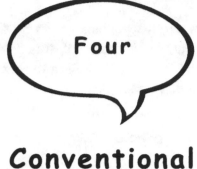

Four

# Conventional Treatments: Medications

If you are taking your child to see the doctor because of symptoms of ear infection such as fever and ear pain, your first line of treatment is most likely going to be medications, both to relieve the immediate symptoms and to treat the infection. In dispensing medications for your child, a delicate balancing act occurs, both for your doctor and you. You want to ease your child's discomfort, but you do not want to give unnecessary medicines that may not help the infection resolve. You may instinctively feel that it is important to do something, but in some cases it may be more prudent to monitor your child and allow the infection to end on its own.

Learning more about the medications commonly used to treat ear infections will give you a better understanding of why each of these medications is used, their potential risks and benefits, and what situations are appropriate for their use. Such information will help you to make more informed decisions with your doctor.

# Antibiotics

Antibiotics are the most widely prescribed first-line treatment for ear infections. Bacterial infections—on their own or coupled with viral infections—are estimated to cause the majority of cases of acute suppurative otitis media (AOM) and nearly one third of cases of otitis media with effusion (OME). Antibiotics can be very effective in treating bacterial infections; however, there is currently a great deal of debate about how frequently antibiotics should be prescribed and under what circumstances their use is most appropriate. To better understand why and how antibiotics have been used, you may find it helpful to learn a little about the history of antibiotics.

## Discovery of Antibiotics

Antibiotics are naturally occurring chemical substances produced by fungi (mold, yeast) or bacteria that inhibit or stop the growth of other bacteria or fungi. The first antibiotic was discovered by accident in 1928 by a Scottish bacteriologist named Alexander Fleming. In experiments to try to kill the bacterium *Staphylococcus aureus* (commonly called staph), Fleming tested various substances against staph growing on plates in his laboratory. If the substance had no effect, the plates were washed clean before being used again for tests with a different substance. On one occasion, however, the plates had not been soaked in detergent and Fleming noticed some mold growing on the surface. The staph around the mold was dead, and Fleming concluded that some substance in the mold had properties that could kill the bacteria. The mold on the plate was *Penicillium notatum,* so Fleming named the bacteria-killing (antibiotic) substance penicillin.

Ten years later, two researchers, Howard Florey and Ernst Chain, discovered how to purify the penicillin from the mold so that it could be used to treat patients. By 1942 they were able to make large quantities of penicillin, and the medicine was used for the first time on a large scale to treat victims of a fire that broke out in a nightclub in Boston. At that time severe burns usually led to death from infection, but the use of penicillin helped save the lives of hundreds of victims of the fire. In 1945 Fleming, Florey, and Chain were awarded the Nobel Prize for the discovery of penicillin. Chemical modifications of penicillin still form the basis of many antibiotics made today.

Since their discovery, antibiotics have proved invaluable for treating serious illnesses including rheumatic fever, tuberculosis, kidney infections, and pneumonia. Effective treatment of bacterial infections has saved countless lives; during the first twenty years of their use alone, antibiotics were estimated to have increased life expectancy in the United States by ten years.

## Overuse of Antibiotics

The National Center for Infectious Diseases recently estimated that 100 million courses of antibiotics are prescribed a year by office-based doctors, and that roughly *half* of these prescriptions are unnecessary. This is partially due to the fact that viral infections often have very similar symptoms to bacterial infections, so it is sometimes difficult for doctors to distinguish what type of infectious agent might be causing illness. As a result, doctors may prescribe antibiotics for viral infections even though antibiotics are not effective against viruses. Moreover, since different antibiotics work against different bacteria, some of the antibiotics that are prescribed—while not being unnecessary—will be ineffective.

The unnecessary and ineffective use of antibiotics has led to the emergence of *antibiotic-resistant* bacteria. When antibiotics are overused, certain strains of bacteria learn how to "outsmart" the antibiotic's killing mechanism. Other, still-sensitive strains of bacteria are killed by the antibiotic, but the resistant strains are able to thrive. So children who have received several courses of a particular antibiotic are more likely to harbor resistant strains of bacteria. If such a child becomes ill subsequent to the antibiotic treatments, it may be harder to treat the new infection because of the high percentage of resistant bacteria. In fact, a key concern for doctors is the treatment of children who have infections caused by resistant strains of the bacterium *Streptococcus pneumoniae*. (*S. pneumoniae* is the most common cause of ear infections, sinus infections, bacterial pneumonia, and bacterial meningitis in children.)

In 1942, every strain of *S. pneumoniae* (there are ninety types) was killed by penicillin, but by the early 1960s a few strains were found to be resistant. During the 1960s, scientists chemically modified penicillin to make it more effective against the resistant bacteria. They also created a new antibiotic using cephalosporin (a substance from a type of mold discovered in a sewer outlet by Italian researcher Giuseppe Brotsu in 1945). But by the mid-1980s, strains of *S. pneumoniae* were also resistant to cephalosporins. Currently, there is only one antibiotic, vancomycin, that is effective against highly resistant strains of *S. pneumoniae*, but it is a very powerful drug that is reserved only for severe cases of infection such as bacterial meningitis. Doctors are concerned that someday soon, strains of *S. pneumoniae* may become resistant to vancomycin as well. In the meantime, vaccinations that are effective against some strains of *S. pneumoniae* are currently being used for high-risk children over two years of age. The American Academy of Pediatrics recently recommended a newer vaccination against *S. pneumoniae* (Prevnar) that can be given to children beginning at two months of age.

For parents and doctors, the best way to reduce the risk of antibiotic-resistant bacteria is to use antibiotics very judiciously, selecting them only for cases in which they are most appropriate. If your child is being treated for an ear infection, you should feel free to tell your doctor that you have concerns about overuse of antibiotics; together you can decide if antibiotics are necessary in your child's case. If your child has already received several courses of antibiotics, there are also steps you can take to help reduce the risk of resistant bacteria. Studies have shown that if antibiotics are stopped for at least six months, the strains of resistant bacteria drop back down to low levels (one study found a decrease from 50 percent down to 5 percent).

## Types of Antibiotics

There are dozens of antibiotics grouped into broad categories based on the substances they are derived from and how they act to kill microorganisms. Five categories of antibiotics are generally used to treat ear infections. The table below provides examples of specific antibiotics in each category. Most of these antibiotics are available in a liquid form (oral antibiotic), some as chewable tablets, and some as injections. The names of the individual antibiotics are listed by their generic (nonbrand) name; the brand name for each drug is capitalized and listed in parentheses. Generic drugs are usually less expensive than their brand name counterparts. (The generic form of an antibiotic should have the same active ingredients as the brand name; only the flavors and inactive ingredients may vary.) However, many of the newer drugs are not yet available in a generic form.

Both the text discussion and table of antibiotics are designed to be a general guide describing how and which antibiotics may be chosen by your doctor to treat your child's ear infection. *It is important to remember that each child's case is different and what is prescribed for one child may not be appropriate for another; also, occurrences of ear infection may be caused by different organisms at different times in the same child.* Medicine is a constantly changing field; new antibiotics are developed all the time and existing antibiotics may be given new indications, treatment schedules, and/or released in different dosages. Thus, one medication may have been prescribed for your older child a few years ago, but a different medication or one in a different dosage schedule may be prescribed now for his brother or sister. Moreover, bacterial resistance to antibiotics changes over time and varies by geographic location, and this also affects the choice of an antibiotic. Your doctor takes these factors into account when choosing an antibiotic for your child.

## Decisions About What Type of Antibiotic to Use

Your doctor will try to select the antibiotic that is most effective at killing the bacteria that she suspects is causing the infection. Her choice will be based on whether it is an initial infection, recurrent infection, or a chronic condition. The doctor's selection also depends on your child's age, history of allergic reactions to antibiotics, and whether your child is taking any ongoing medications. The more you know about these considerations, the more input you can offer in decisions about antibiotic treatment.

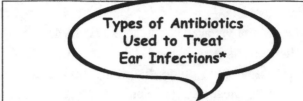

**Types of Antibiotics
Used to Treat
Ear Infections***

<u>Penicillins</u> disrupt the building of bacterial cell walls using a special molecule called beta-lactam; bacteria that are resistant to penicillins produce a protein called beta-lactamase that breaks down this molecule.

amoxicillin (Amoxil, Trimox, Wymox)
- Considered best first choice for treating initial cases of AOM; strong against the three main bacteria implicated in AOM†
- New, more effective twice-daily dosing available
- Absorbed well in digestive tract, few side effects
- Not recommended for children under one month old
- Not good for repeat infections; many bacteria have grown resistant to amoxicillin

amoxicillin-clavulanate (Augmentin)‡
- Often used after amoxicillin has failed; strong against amoxicillin-resistant bacteria
- Not recommended for children under one month old

<u>Cephalosporins</u> disrupt bacterial cell wall building, but without the special beta-lactam molecule used by some penicillins so they are more effective against bacteria that are resistant to penicillin; children who are allergic to penicillin may also react to cephalosporins.

cefprozil (Cefzil)
- Broad spectrum drug, effective on a wide range of bacteria

- Good second choice if amoxicillin has failed; particularly strong against *S. pneumoniae*
- Not recommended for children under six months old

cefixime (Suprax)‡
- Once-a-day dose
- Strong against the three main bacteria implicated in AOM,* but least effective against *S. pneumoniae*
- Good second choice if the first antibiotic tried was strong against *S. pneumoniae* but failed
- Not recommended for children under 6 months old

ceftriaxone (Rocephin)‡
- Given by injection into the arm muscle (intramuscular)
- Newer drug, recommended as second line of treatment; strong against amoxicillin-resistant bacteria

cefuroxime axetil (Ceftin)‡
- Newer drug, recommended as a second line of treatment; strong against amoxicillin-resistant bacteria
- Not recommended for children under three months old

There are numerous other cephalosporins used to treat ear infections, including cefpodoxime proxetil (Vantin), cefaclor (Ceclor), and ceftibuten (Cedax).

Macrolides keep bacteria from producing proteins so they cannot reproduce.

azithromycin (Zithromax)‡
- Once-a-day dose for only 5 days
- Strong against the three main bacteria implicated in AOM,* but less effective against *H. influenzae*

- Used if child is allergic to penicillins,
  cephalosporins, and sulfonamides (see below)
- Not recommended for children under 6 months

**clarithromycin (Biaxin)‡**
- Strong against the three main bacteria implicated
  in AOM,* but less effective against *H. influenzae*
- Good choice if child is allergic to penicillins,
  cephalosporins, and sulfonamides (see below)
- Not recommended for children under 6 months

**Sulfonamides and sulfa combination drugs** are sulfur-containing antibiotics. Several cautions are connected with sulfas, so children using these medications should be closely monitored:
- Sulfas can lower the body's white blood cell count,
  lowering resistance to other infections.
- Sulfas need to be given with lots of liquid to keep
  the medication from crystallizing in the kidneys.
- Sulfas can sensitize skin to the sun, so children should
  avoid sun or use sunscreen protection when necessary.

**sulfisoxazole acetyl (Gantrisin)‡**
- In the past was used as onetime daily dose over
  several months for prevention, but now because
  of antibiotic resistance, once daily preventive
  antibiotics are not recommended
- Not recommended for children under 6 months old

**trimethoprim-sulfamethoxazole (Bactrim, Cotrim, Septra, Sulfatrim)**
- Used only if others not effective; not for prolonged
  or repeated use

- Not recommended for children under 2 months old

erythromycin-sulfisoxazole (Pediazole, Eryzole)
- Requires 3–4 daily doses
- Not recommended for children under 2 months old

*This list is not comprehensive but includes many of the antibiotics most commonly prescribed by doctors for AOM. There are numerous other antibiotics used to treat ear infections and new ones are under development.

† The three main types of bacteria most commonly found in cases of AOM are *Streptococcus pneumoniae, Haemophilus influenzae, and Moraxella catarrhalis.*

‡ Denotes antibiotics that are *not* available in a generic form.

### Initial Infections

As we have said before, it is difficult to predict exactly which bacteria may be causing an ear infection, but the majority of cases of acute suppurative otitis media (AOM) are thought to be caused by one of three bacteria: *Streptococcus pneumoniae, Hemophilus influenzae, and Moraxella catarrhalis.* These bacteria are also found in approximately one third of cases of otitis media with effusion (OME). Amoxicillin is therefore usually the first choice for treating an initial case of ear infection because it has few side effects and is effective against these three bacteria (although it is not quite as strong against *H. influenzae* as it is against the other two bacteria). The use of a higher dose given twice daily, rather than a dose given three times a day, has been approved by the U.S. Food and Drug Administration (FDA) to increase the effectiveness of amoxicillin.

If your child's symptoms do not improve in three to four days after taking amoxicillin, it means the antibiotic is not working, and your doctor may want to try another antibiotic. Alternatives could include an antibiotic that is more effective against *H. influenzae* (such as cefixime); one that is strong against a wide variety of bacteria (such as cefprozil); one that has been shown to be effective against bacteria that are resistant to amoxicillin (such as amoxicillin clavulanate), or using the new recommended combination of amoxicillin and Augmentin.

### Recurrent Infections

If your child has had several episodes of AOM or OME in a season, amoxicillin would not be used to treat subsequent cases because of the likelihood of the infection being caused by bacteria that are resistant to this antibiotic. At that point, the doctor may consider using an antibiotic that is effective against bacteria that are resistant to amoxicillin (such as amoxicillin clavulanate or a cephalosporin).

In a few cases, if your child is heading into another winter season and is already showing a similar pattern of repeat infections, your doctor might want to try a *preventive* course of low-dose antibiotics. Sulfisoxazole acetyl (Gantrisin) was developed specifically for prevention but has some adverse effects. In general, long-term use (for periods of three to six months) of preventive antibiotics (prophylaxis) is no longer routinely advised because of the increasing incidence of resistant bacteria.

### Chronic Infection

For cases of chronic suppurative otitis media in which the ear continues to drain pus (called otorrhea) through a perforated eardrum, *topical* antibiotics are used. Topical means they are applied directly to the site of the infection through ear drops in the ear canal. These antibiotics belong to different families than the oral antibiotics used to treat AOM and OME. The only treatment currently approved by the FDA is ofloxacin otic (Floxin Otic) solution. Studies have shown it to be safe and effective during a ten-day course. Another topical medication, Cortisporin Otic (a combination of an antibiotic and steroid), is also used by some doctors for this condition, although it has not received FDA approval for this use. Long-term use of otic drops is not recommended because researchers are still studying to what degree such use might affect functioning of the inner ear.

### Age of Your Child

All of the antibiotics given to children for ear infections are considered safe for children over six months of age. However, if your child is under six months old, only certain oral antibiotics will be considered for selection, including:

- amoxicillin and amoxicillin-clavulanate: safe for children one month and older

- erythromycin-sulfisoxazole and trimethoprim-sulfisoxazole: safe for children two months and older

Oral antibiotics are not considered appropriate treatment for infants under one month old, and rarely will a doctor prescribe an oral antibiotic for a child under two months. Most often children under two months will be given an intravenous antibiotic if the medication is required, or will be observed without the use of antibiotics.

*Other Medications Currently Being Taken*

You should always inform your doctor of any other medications—prescription, over-the-counter, and alternative—that your child is currently taking because antibiotics can interact with other drugs, particularly asthma medicines and antihistamines. For example, clarithromycin (one of the macrolides), tends to interact with medicines more frequently than other antibiotics. In most cases, your doctor will be able to select antibiotics with the least risk of interaction and find ways for your child to take antibiotics along with his ongoing medication.

*History of Allergic Reactions to Antibiotics*

If your child has taken any antibiotics in the past and had an allergic reaction, you should inform your doctor before she starts making decisions about antibiotic choice. If your child is allergic to penicillin, an antibiotic from the macrolides family—such as azithromycin—or a sulfonamide would be used. Children who are allergic to antibiotics from the penicillin family are also frequently allergic to cephalosporins as well, so antibiotics from this family may not be used.

If your child is taking antibiotics, ask your doctor to explain the signs of allergic reaction for the specific antibiotic being prescribed, and get instructions for what to do if you notice such signs. Typical allergic reactions could include raised, red welts on the skin (hives), difficulty breathing, or vomiting. These symptoms are different than the more mild side effects of antibiotics (discussed below). Other more serious allergic reactions include anaphylactic shock (loss of consciousness) and adverse effects on the cardiovascular, central nervous, endocrine, or respiratory systems; these types of reactions are very serious and *very* uncommon in children.

If you notice any signs of possible allergic reaction, you should stop the antibiotic treatment (most symptoms subside once the treatment is stopped) and contact your doctor immediately. She will advise you on how to treat the reaction and also prescribe an alternative antibiotic.

## Side Effects of Antibiotics

You should be aware of the possible side effects of antibiotics; side effects are different from an allergic reaction (see above). Side effects are usually mild and subside as the treatment course ends. Although side effects can vary depending on the antibiotic, the most common ones are diarrhea, yeast infections, and skin rashes.

Such conditions may warrant discontinuing the medication, but only after discussing the situation with your doctor. She may advise you to stop treatment and prescribe an alternative antibiotic.

### Diarrhea

Oral antibiotics do not go directly to the site of the infection in the middle ear; they are absorbed through the bloodstream and can interact with microorganisms in the digestive tract. This interaction can sometimes cause diarrhea, abdominal discomfort, or a little nausea. You should encourage your child to drink plenty of fluids to help combat the dehydration that can accompany diarrhea. The occurrence of diarrhea is also reduced by giving the antibiotic with food. Some parents also give their children yogurt with live cultures (*Lactobacillus acidophilus*) to replace some of the beneficial bacteria in the intestines and reduce the risk of diarrhea.

### Yeast Infections

Sometimes beneficial bacteria can also be killed by antibiotics, resulting in yeast infections in the vagina and in the skin around the diaper area in babies. You should change your child's diaper frequently to keep the genitalia and buttocks area clean and dry. The *Lactobacillus acidophilus* in yogurt (see above) may also help to diminish the effects of yeast infection.

### Skin Rashes

Mild skin rashes can also appear, usually patches of red skin or raised bumps; estimated to occur in about 3 to 4 percent of cases. These rashes are in contrast to hives or large welts, which generally signal an allergic reaction. Benadryl (diphenhydramine hydrochloride) can be given for these skin reactions.

## Instructions for Antibiotic Use

When you receive your antibiotics you should also receive specific information about dosage, storage, and possible side effects. You should review these instructions with your doctor or pharmacist to make sure the information is clear. Feel free to ask questions if there is anything you do not understand. *Proper administration of antibiotics is central to their effectiveness.*

### Dosage

Many oral antibiotics are now given twice a day (instead of the three or four times a day that was required in the past). The number of days an antibiotic is necessary for ear infections is controversial and varies with the medication chosen. One of the most important things you can do if

## A Personal Experience:
## A New Infection

Diane was disappointed that her three-year-old, Nicole, was sick again nine days after her last doctor's visit. Her daughter, once again, had ear pain and for the sixth time the pediatrician told them that Nicole had an ear infection.

Diane couldn't understand how a new infection had followed so swiftly after the last one. During the visit, the doctor asked her a few questions about how the week had been and how Nicole had been feeling. Diane had been pleased when Nicole had begun to feel much better only two days after she had started the medicine, so Diane had sent Nicole back to day care. The doctor inquired as to whether Nicole had completed the full course of antibiotics. Diane acknowledged that it was difficult to keep up with all the dosages after Nicole was back at day care, as there was no one available to administer the afternoon dose. Since Nicole had begun feeling much better and didn't like the taste of the medicine, Diane had discontinued the medicine four days after starting it.

The pediatrician explained how stopping the medication before its course was completed might be the cause of Nicole's infection returning so quickly. He stressed that it was important to complete the full dosage for the prescribed length of time in order for the antibiotic to work fully. They agreed to try using medication with a different dosage schedule the next time (perhaps an antibiotic that can be given fewer times a day or for fewer days) and also to try a medication that tastes better.

using antibiotics is to follow the prescribed dosage precisely. It can be challenging to follow the treatment schedule; your child may not like the taste of the antibiotic and it can be hard to remember to give the doses over the usual ten days during the hectic family routines. If the infection does not clear and your child did not get the proper dosage, it will be difficult to determine whether the antibiotic failed due to insufficient dosage or because of the occurrence of resistant strains of bacteria.

In addition, you should check whether the antibiotic needs to be given on its own, with food, or with other liquids. Appropriate administering will ensure more effective treatment.

### *Storage*

Usually antibiotics are given in oral form to treat ear infections. The liquid is slowly absorbed into the bloodstream through the stomach or intestinal wall. Many of these liquids need to be refrigerated, as they will not be effective if left at room temperature. A few oral antibiotics— including azithromycin and cefixime—do not need to be refrigerated.

Amoxicillin and amoxicillin-clavulanate are also available as chewable tablets. The tablets do not need to be refrigerated and may be more convenient if you are traveling or taking your child to day care or school. Older children often prefer chewable tablets to taking the liquid.

## Decisions About Whether to Use Antibiotics

The information available about antibiotic use and ear infections is full of contradictions. Several studies have shown that treatment of ear infections with antibiotics helps to speed the recovery process; 90 to 95 percent of children get better after one course of antibiotics. *However, other studies have shown that 70 to 80 percent of cases of ear infection resolve on their own without any antibiotic treatment.* One review of published studies on the topic concluded that clinical trials have not proved antibiotic effectiveness for ear infections. Other recent studies suggest that antibiotic treatments of only five to seven days may be just as effective as ten days. Concerns about antibiotic-resistant bacteria have also entered into the debate about the use of antibiotics for ear infections. Some members of the medical community are recommending more large-scale studies that compare the effects of antibiotics with that of monitoring and observation in treating children with ear infections to determine whether antibiotics should continue to be used as a first-line treatment. In the meantime, antibiotics are still the most widely used treatment for ear infections.

As a parent there are a few factors to consider in deciding with your doctor whether or not to use antibiotics; these factors vary somewhat depending on whether your child has been diagnosed with AOM or OME. If your doctor has not specified her diagnosis, ask her to do so before discussing antibiotic use.

### Treating AOM

If your child has an initial case of AOM, with ear pain and fever, and has not previously received several courses of antibiotics, then antibiotic treatment is a reasonable choice, since the majority of AOM is thought to be caused by bacterial infections. However, if your child is not experiencing a lot of discomfort from ear pain or fever, an option you may want to consider is to use acetaminophen (e.g., Tylenol) to alleviate the symptoms, and wait two to three days to see if the infection will resolve on its own. If the symptoms persist or become more severe, you should consult with your doctor about whether to proceed with antibiotic treatment.

If your child is having recurrent infections, and has already been given several courses of antibiotics, it is a good idea to work with your doctor to try to address any potential risk factors or underlying causes of infection (see Chapter 2) before continuing with repeated rounds of antibiotics.

### Treating OME

If your child has OME, it is more difficult to predict what the infecting bacteria may be, because a much wider range of bacteria may be responsible (see Chapter 2). In addition, only 30 percent of cases of OME are thought to be caused by bacteria, so antibiotics may not be the best first line of treatment for OME.

In 1994, the Agency for Health Care Policy and Research (AHCPR) (part of the U.S. Department of Health and Human Services) published guidelines for treating OME in otherwise healthy children aged one to three years based on a review of research and on the opinions of a panel of experts convened to discuss the topic. The group concluded that monitoring and observation is a viable treatment option for OME for up to three months if no hearing impairment is detected. In addition, treatment should include efforts to address risk factors or underlying causes. However, they also stated that antibiotic treatment is a reasonable alternative.

If your child has ear fluid that lasts beyond three months and there are signs of hearing impairment of 20 dB or more in one ear, many doctors—and parents—may prefer to try at least one course of antibiotic treatment before considering surgical interventions.

## Discussing Antibiotic Use with Your Doctor

Surveys have found that many parents often are misinformed about antibiotic use. Findings from one study revealed that most parents think antibiotics are sometimes or always necessary to treat ear infections. While the majority of parents are aware of the problems associated with overuse of antibiotics, many still call their doctor requesting that antibiotics be prescribed. Some parents even give their child antibiotics at home without first consulting a doctor, a practice that is strongly discouraged.

As a result, many doctors have learned that parents expect and want antibiotics to be prescribed; some even think it is central to providing patient satisfaction. These doctors are much more likely to give a bacterial diagnosis and prescribe antibiotics.

To avoid such misunderstandings, the best thing you can do is to communicate openly with your doctor.

- Tell your doctor that you do not automatically expect antibiotics to be prescribed for your child.
- Let your doctor know that you want antibiotics to be used only if she feels it is necessary and appropriate for your child's case.
- If you have concerns about overuse of antibiotics and the risk of your child developing antibiotic-resistant bacteria, you should discuss them with your doctor.
- If your doctor is ready to prescribe antibiotics, ask her to explain specifically why she is recommending them, what her diagnosis is, and if there are other treatment options.

Opening up lines of communication can increase understanding (and decrease confusion) between you and your child's doctor.

# Other Medications

Other conventional medicines have been used to treat ear infections, including analgesics, antihistamines, decongestants, and steroids. While you may find some of these medications helpful in relieving your child's symptoms, they are not effective in killing the organisms that may be causing the infection. In addition, antihistamines, decongestants, and steroids have side effects that may outweigh their potential benefits, and none of these three medication types have been recommended for use in the AHCPR guidelines (see page 98) for treating OME.

## Analgesics

Analgesics are medications that help to control pain, reduce inflammation, or lower fever in the body. Two types of analgesics are sometimes used to manage the fever and ear pain associated with ear infections: acetaminophen (Tylenol, Panadol), an aspirin substitute, and nonsteroidal anti-inflammatory drugs, such as ibuprofen (Motrin, Advil). Analgesics may help your child to feel better, but they do not speed the recovery process or cure the infection. Ear drops that use a painkilling medication are also available, although overuse of these drops can mask symptoms.

Although research suggests that fever actually helps the body's immune system respond better (the higher temperature facilitates better functioning of the lymph cells that fight infection), giving your child an analgesic will make him more comfortable and relieve his pain. It is not necessary to contact your doctor immediately for a moderate-grade fever (102° F or below), but if the following situations exist, speak to your doctor right away:

- The fever persists or gets higher

- Your child is younger than three months of age and has a rectal temperature of 100.4° F or higher

- Your child is between three and thirty-six months of age and has a rectal temperature of 102.2° F or higher

### Risks of Analgesics

Aspirin is never prescribed for children because of its potentially harmful effects in treatment of viral infections. Such effects can include vomiting, swelling of the brain, and dysfunction of the liver (together this collection of symptoms is known as Reye's syndrome).

If you use acetaminophen, you should only give your child a product that is made specifically for children, and you should follow the dosage instructions precisely (based on your child's age or, ideally, have your doctor prescribe a dose based on your child's weight); higher doses or more frequent doses than the recommended amount can be harmful. In addition, you should check the labels of any over-the-counter cough and cold medications that you give to your child. Many of these are combination medications and may contain acetaminophen, so you could inadvertently give your child too high a dose.

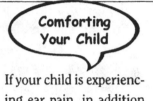

**Comforting Your Child**

If your child is experiencing ear pain, in addition to using an analgesic, you can help make your child more comfortable by applying a warm washcloth to the sore ear (some children prefer a cool cloth). You may also want to try an appropriate homeopathic medicine after consulting with your doctor first (see Chapter 6). For more tips on comforting your child, also see Chapter 7.

## Antihistamines and Decongestants

Both antihistamines and decongestants have been routinely prescribed to treat allergies or colds accompanying an ear infection. However, studies have shown that neither medication improves eustachian tube or middle ear function or affects the course of an ear infection. The AHCPR guidelines for treating OME (see page 98) specifically discourage the use of antihistamines and decongestants, citing no benefits and the possible harm to children through the side effects of such medications. (Moreover, over-the-counter cough and cold medicines that contain antihistamines and decongestants have not been shown to be very effective in relieving symptoms of the common cold in children younger than five years.)

Antihistamines are drugs that are principally used to relieve allergy symptoms such as watery eyes and runny nose. Histamines are natural substances in the body released during allergic reactions that cause dilation of blood vessels or itchiness on the skin. When antihistamines are absorbed into the bloodstream, they block the histamines from dilating the blood vessels, which helps reduce congestion in the nose. Antihistamines do not cure the allergic reaction; they simply relieve the symptoms. Antihistamines can be bought over the counter; some common brand names of antihistamines are Benadryl and Chlor-Trimeton. The most common side effects from such medications are drowsiness, shakiness, blurred vision, and upset stomach.

Decongestants relieve stuffiness and may make your child feel more comfortable, but they do nothing to stop infection. Common over-the-counter decongestants include Sudafed and Dimetapp. In some children decongestants act as a stimulant; common side effects include restlessness, agitation, and irritability. In other children, decongestants cause drowsiness.

### Risks of Antihistamines and Decongestants

In addition to the side effects noted above, antihistamines and decongestants can alter blood pressure and damage the tiny hairs (cilia) in the membranes of the nose and eustachian tube; these hairs help move bacteria and fluid out of the middle ear and the nasal cavity.

### Alternatives to Antihistamines and Decongestants

If your child is suffering from runny nose and congestion accompanying an ear infection, it may be difficult for you to stop using antihistamines or decongestants. However, there are other ways that you can give your child some relief. Saline (saltwater) drops applied in the nostrils and then sucked out by a bulb aspirator help thin out mucus in the nasal passages. Drops can be applied several times a day. Other simple comforts include elevating your child's head, giving him lots of fluids, and helping him to blow his nose. For infants and young children who cannot blow their nose, a bulb aspirator can be used to gently suck out the excess mucus. You may also want to try a homeopathic medicine designed specifically to relieve congestion, after consulting with your doctor (see Chapter 6).

## Steroids

Steroids are chemical substances produced by the body that help to regulate its functions (for example, stimulation of bone growth and maturation of the reproductive organs). Certain types of steroids—corticosteroids—have a strong anti-inflammatory effect and are prescribed as medications to treat various conditions; the steroid cortisone, for example, is used to treat rheumatoid arthritis. Corticosteroids have also been used on a short-term basis to treat chronic suppurative otitis media, certain complications of ear infections (such as labyrinthitis), and inner ear disorders, usually in combination with an antibiotic.

Researchers have studied the effects of corticosteroids in shrinking swollen tissue in the eustachian tube and in thinning fluid in the middle ear, but they have found no evidence that corticosteroids help to clear middle ear fluid. Some study results looking at steroid therapy—alone or in combination with antibiotics—to treat OME have also been inconclusive, although other studies support the use of steroids in treating ear infections. The AHCPR guidelines for treating OME (see page 98) do not recommend use of steroid treatment at the present time.

### Risks of Steroids

The potential side effects of steroids include agitation, behavior changes, sleeplessness, increased appetite, and weight gain. In some cases, steroid treatments have been found to actually enhance the strength of viruses in acute infections. Rare complications include digestive disorders, chest pain, and Cushing's disease—overfunctioning of the adrenal gland, which leads to increased steroid production in the body.

# Five

# Conventional
# Treatments: Surgery

Most parents of children with ear infections will never need to consider surgical treatments for their children, because 70 to 80 percent of ear infections resolve on their own without any treatment. An additional 15 to 20 percent of cases respond to medical treatment in a matter of days or weeks. Therefore, only in a small percentage of cases will surgical procedures be considered.

If your child has a history of recurrent ear infections and has *not* responded to medical (nonsurgical) treatments or to preventive measures, then your doctor will most likely refer you to an ear, nose, and throat (ENT) specialist (otolaryngologist) for further evaluation. However, it is important to remember that referral to an ENT doctor does *not* automatically mean your child needs surgery. The ENT doctor will look for specific indicators to assess whether surgery would be appropriate for your child. (The American Academy of Otolaryngology–Head and Neck Surgery has established guidelines with specific indicators for considering surgical procedures for the treatment of ear infections in children.)

In addition, every child's case needs to be considered individually and as a parent you can play a valuable part in discussing surgical treatment. If you understand what each procedure involves (including follow-up care and potential complications) and learn the benefits as well as the limitations of each type of surgery, you can make more informed choices about whether surgery is the best option for your child.

If you decide to go forward with surgery for your child, you should also be reassured that the surgical procedures used to treat ear infections are safe, simple, and effective when used in the appropriate situations. Three types of procedures are generally considered for ear infections:

- Myringotomy (making an incision to drain the fluid from the middle ear), with or without taking a sample of the middle ear fluid to test for the presence of bacteria or viruses. (In tympanocentesis, a thin, hollow needle is used to draw out fluid from the middle ear for testing.) Myringotomy is not commonly used without the insertion of tympanostomy tubes.
- Myringotomy with insertion of tympanostomy tubes (small metal or plastic tubes inserted through the eardrum to allow drainage of fluid from the middle ear and to keep the middle ear ventilated)
- Adenoidectomy (removal of the adenoids located at the back of the throat near the nasal passage)

## Myringotomy and Tympanocentesis

Myringotomy and tympanocentesis are procedures used to drain fluid from the middle ear. In myringotomy, a tiny cut is made in the eardrum and the collected fluid and pus is allowed to drain out of the ear canal or is gently suctioned out and may possibly be sent for testing for the presence of bacteria or viruses. In tympanocentesis, a thin, hollow needle is inserted into the middle ear cavity to draw out some of the fluid to be tested to identify the infecting organism (such as a virus or bacterium). The results of the test or culture determine whether antibiotics are an appropriate treatment and also which antibiotics would be most effective at stopping the infection.

## When Are Myringotomy and Tympanocentesis Considered?

Your ENT doctor may recommend myringotomy or tympanocentesis if your child is less than thirty days old or has any of the following conditions:

- An unusually severe case of acute suppurative otitis media (AOM) characterized by intense ear pain, high fever, increasing hearing loss, or vertigo (feeling of dizziness)
- Frequent repeat episodes of AOM (more than three episodes in six months or more than four episodes in one year) that have not responded to two or more antibiotics or to treatments that address underlying factors such as allergic conditions or environmental factors
- Recurrent otitis media with effusion (OME) (fluid lasting longer than three months) that has not responded to consecutive antibiotics or to treatments that address underlying factors such as allergic conditions or environmental factors
- Immunosuppression, such as what happens during chemotherapy treatment for cancer

## How Are Myringotomy and Tympanocentesis Performed?

### Myringotomy

Myringotomy without tube placement may be performed in the doctor's office without anesthesia; some doctors use a local anesthesia applied to the eardrum five to ten minutes before the procedure. In some cases, your child may require sedation in preparation for this short but painful procedure. The incision (cut) in the eardrum is made with a tiny surgical knife (scalpel), and is carefully done to avoid any injury to the floor of the middle ear or to the bones (ossicles) of the middle ear. If the fluid is thin and clear, a pinprick incision is adequate to drain the ear; for buildup of pus or thicker effusions, a slightly larger incision is needed. A suction tip may be used to remove the fluid or it may be allowed to drain on its own.

It is very important that your child does not move during this procedure. The doctor will want to secure your child in a cloth wrapping (called a papoose) to keep her from moving during the procedure. You can sit by your child's side to comfort and reassure her during the surgery. At the start of the procedure, your child will feel a slight pressure, then a momentary pain when the incision is made. She will then feel the suction as fluid is drawn out and hear a loud sucking noise. Your child should feel better immediately after the procedure; the pressure on her eardrum will be relieved, her middle ear will be aerated, and her hearing may be more clear.

### Tympanocentesis

In tympanocentesis, a puncture is made in the eardrum (myringotomy), then a hollow needle is used to draw out and collect the fluid. The sample of fluid is then tested for the presence of viruses or bacteria.

The procedure for myringotomy and tympanocentesis is actually quite similar; the only real difference is that in tympanocentesis the collected fluid is sent for analysis.

## What Is the Follow-up for Myringotomy and Tympanocentesis?

### Myringotomy

The cut in your child's eardrum will heal rapidly, usually in three days. However, her ear may continue to drain a little fluid or pus during and after the cut's healing; this discharge is called *otorrhea*. The main thing you should do to care for your child after the surgery is to keep her ear dry and clean. Clean your hands before touching her ear, use sterile cotton pads to wipe away any discharge, and try to keep your child from touching the discharge.

Many doctors will schedule a follow-up visit for twenty-four to forty-eight hours after the surgery to make sure the incision is healing well. One month later, the doctor may recheck the ear to make sure there are no signs of infection and to see that the discharge from the ear has stopped.

### Tympanocentesis

The eardrum will heal rapidly, but discharge from the ear may continue for a few days. Follow-up care for the ear is similar to that of simple myringotomy. In addition, when results of the tested ear fluid come back (usually in one to two days), your doctor will schedule a follow-up visit to discuss what antibiotic treatment would be most appropriate—if at all—based on the microorganisms identified in the culture. If the decision is made to use antibiotics, your doctor will prescribe the medication and check back with you in three days to see whether your child's symptoms have subsided, a sign that the antibiotic is working.

## What Are the Potential Complications of Myringotomy and Tympanocentesis?

Myringotomy and tympanocentesis may cause slight scarring of the eardrum (tympanosclerosis); such scarring is not frequent, is generally very mild, and does not affect hearing. The other potential complication is infection at the site of the incision in the eardrum. However, this happens even more rarely and can be treated effectively with antibiotic drops applied in the ear.

More serious complications are extremely rare. The main risk as with any invasive procedure is if the procedure is not properly performed. Your doctor will advise you of how the procedure is performed and will discuss potential complications. This process is part of the informed consent process that is standard practice in medicine.

## What Are the Benefits and Limitations of Myringotomy and Tympanocentesis?

### Myringotomy

Myringotomy is effective for *temporarily* draining the ear; it immediately relieves pressure on the eardrum and restores normal ventilation to the middle ear. However, its effects are not long-term; fluid can accumulate again, and in some cases several myringotomies may be necessary.

For the past twenty years, myringotomy has not been commonly performed in the United States as a single procedure; instead it is performed in conjunction with insertion of tympanostomy tubes (see page 112). With the rise in antibiotic therapy, many training programs for pediatricians stopped teaching the procedure. At present, it is mainly used by ENT doctors to temporarily relieve pressure on the eardrum if a child  is seriously ill and has not responded to initial antibiotic treatment.

### Tympanocentesis

When the middle ear fluid is collected and analyzed, it can be very useful for making treatment decisions about children who have acute and repeated ear infections and who have responded poorly to antibiotics. A middle ear fluid specimen is the best way to determine the infectious agent and to decide if antibiotic treatment is appropriate. This information can greatly reduce the use of antibiotics by identifying cases of ear infection that are *not* caused by bacteria.

At the present time tympanocentesis is not commonly performed. The American Academy of Otolaryngology–Head and Neck Surgery recommends that tympanocentesis only be performed by an ENT doctor because of the risk of possible serious complications. However, some doctors feel that the risks of tympanocentesis are minimal and that the procedure should be taught to pediatricians and family practitioners and used more frequently to better diagnose and treat ear infections and to avoid unnecessary use of antibiotics. Recently, a number of ENT doctors have agreed to serve on a national faculty in a continuing medical education course to train community-based primary care physicians in the technique of office-based tympanocentesis.

# Myringotomy with Insertion of Tympanostomy Tubes

Myringotomy with insertion of tympanostomy tubes involves making an incision in the eardrum, then inserting a tiny tube through the eardrum (tympanic membrane) into the middle ear. The tubes (sometimes called grommets, pressure-equalization tubes, or PETs) stay in place for a variable period of time, with an average time of nine months. The tubes allow fluid to drain out of the ear, provide ventilation or aeration for the middle ear, and improve hearing. Tympanostomy tubes are made of a variety of materials and come in a variety of shapes and sizes. Different designs are intended to ease insertion or removal of the tube or to prolong the time the tube stays in the eardrum.

## When Is Insertion of Tympanostomy Tubes Considered?

Your ENT doctor will review your child's history of middle ear problems and other illnesses, conduct a physical exam looking at the eardrum and the middle ear, and use audiometry and tympanometry tests to check hearing and functioning of the ear. The doctor may recommend tympanostomy surgery if your child has any of the following conditions:

- Persistent or chronic OME—when fluid persists longer than three months and hearing loss is over 20 decibels in one ear (see Chapter 3), or there are signs of language and speech delays
- Recurrent AOM (more than three episodes in six months or more than four episodes in one year) that has not responded to at least two different courses of antibiotics,

one course specifically for resistant bacteria (antibiotic use is discussed in Chapter 4)

- Severe AOM characterized by signs of potential complications such as mastoiditis (see Chapter 1)
- Existing conditions such as a cleft palate or Down syndrome in which the eustachian tube does not provide adequate drainage for the middle ear (see Chapter 2)

## Discussing Insertion of Tympanostomy Tubes with Your Doctor

Because tympanostomy is a surgical procedure requiring the use of general anesthesia, it is usually considered only as a final option after medical (nonsurgical) treatments and preventive measures have failed. However, tympanostomy has become a routine procedure in the United States; it is estimated that 670,000 procedures are performed every year.

If your ENT doctor recommends the procedure for your child, ask her to explain specifically why she is suggesting it, so that you will be clear about the reasons. If the doctor has found significant hearing impairment, signs of speech or language delays, or symptoms of possible complications, it is probably best to go forward with the surgery. It is important that you still take the time to discuss the procedure with your doctor, asking questions and seeking additional information until you feel satisfied it is the best decision for your child.

In addition, you should be aware that there are circumstances where it would be prudent to wait a little longer before moving forward with surgery or where other options might be more feasible. If you think your child's case is characterized by any of the following situations, you can discuss with your doctor whether it may be feasible to hold off on surgery.

- If your child has OME in only one ear at a time, and has very mild hearing impairment and normal language development, then it may be best to continue monitoring her and postpone a decision about surgery. Remember that 60 percent of OME goes away on its own by three months, and 85 percent resolves within six months.
- If your child is having frequent episodes of AOM but the infections are not severe or the infections are responding to antibiotics, then delaying or deciding against surgery can be considered.
- If the spring season is pending, you may decide to postpone surgery until the fall because there is a chance your child may not get new ear infections in the spring. You can discuss the issue again with your doctor during the next winter season if your child continues to get recurrent infections and does not respond to preventive efforts or medications.

In the end, thoughtful decision making by both you and your doctor can ensure that tympanostomy will be used only if it is found necessary after careful evaluation of all of the aspects of your child's situation.

## How Are Tympanostomy Tubes Inserted?

Tympanostomy is performed in a hospital under general anesthesia. Each doctor and each hospital has its own plan for preoperative and postoperative care for your child. You should review what to expect on the day of your child's surgery with your child's doctor or nurse (for example, at

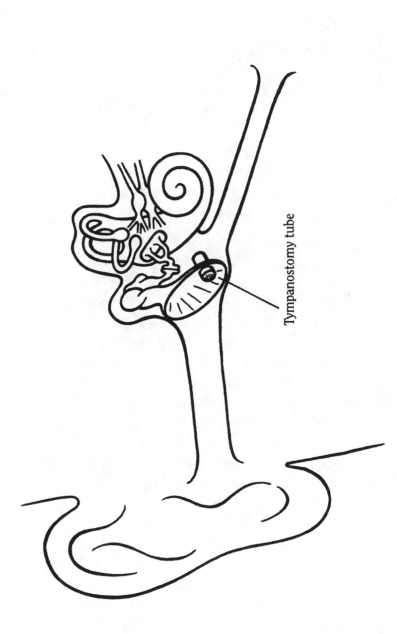

Tympanostomy tube

FIGURE FOUR  Cross-section of the ear showing a tympanostomy tube in place

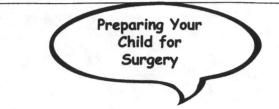

Preparing Your Child for Surgery

The following suggestions provide a few ideas for ways to prepare your child for having surgery. You can decide which of the measures may be most appropriate for your child, depending on his personality and age.

- Read books with your child about trips to the hospital, such as *Curious George Goes to the Hospital* or *A Visit to the Sesame Street Hospital,* which describes Grover's tour of the hospital before his tonsillectomy (see Resources, page 227).
- Play games about the hospital in the weeks prior to the surgery, such as letting your child put pretend tubes in his teddy bear's ears.
- Plan a visit to the hospital beforehand and let your child go to the cafeteria or gift shop to get some ice cream or other special treat. Some hospitals may arrange special tours for parents and children before the surgery so they can see the operating and/or recovery rooms.
- Prepare for the surgery as a special day or outing for you and your child. She can select a favorite book, toy, blanket, or small game to bring with her. She can pick out what clothes she wants to wear to go to the hospital. Older children might like to bring a small journal and write about some of the things they see at the hospital while they are waiting.

- You can explain in simple terms what will happen on the day of the surgery. The doctor or hospital staff may be able to provide you with a brochure or a video about the procedure.

what point you will be able to take your child home). Usually, the procedures most hospitals follow will be similar to those described here.

Because of the use of anesthesia, your child should not eat or drink anything for eight hours prior to the surgery. You will need to arrive at the hospital a few hours before the scheduled surgery. Feel free to bring a few favorite books, toys, or games to help keep your child happy and occupied during the wait. A nurse will bring some paperwork for you to fill out and will check your child's vital signs (temperature, pulse, blood pressure). The anesthesiologist will also meet with you to explain how the anesthesia will be administered (usually by breathing gas through a mask).

Before the operation, your ENT doctor (who will perform the surgery) will stop by to see how you and your child are doing and answer any last-minute questions you might have. When the hospital staff is ready to start the procedure, you can accompany your child as far as the waiting area outside of the operating room. The surgery takes about ten to fifteen minutes: your child receives the anesthesia, the incision is made, the tubes are inserted, and antibiotic drops are applied in the ear. The doctor will usually come to see you immediately afterward to let you know how the surgery went.

Your child will be brought to a recovery room where you can rejoin her. She may be a little groggy from the anesthesia and should rest in bed for a few hours. Initially the nurse will encourage her to have a few sips of water; after two hours she can try more fluids, then a little solid food. The nurse will also review with you instructions about care for your child in the days following the surgery.

Your child should feel fine once the anesthesia has worn off. The pressure on her eardrum has been relieved and her hearing should be improved.

## What Is the Follow-up for Insertion of Tympanostomy Tubes?

The cut in your child's eardrum will heal around the tube after a few hours, but her ears may continue to drain fluid (otorrhea) for a few days. If the effusion has an increased viscosity (is thicker) and/or if your child is under three years old the drainage may last a little longer.

There are several things you can do to care for your child's ears in the weeks after the surgery.

- **Allow the ear to drain freely.** If there is discharge from your child's ear, do not put cotton plugs into the ear canal; a small piece of sterile cotton gauze may be loosely placed in the ear to absorb drainage and then be removed.
- **Keep the external ear dry and clean.** Use warm water and a sterile pad to clean and dry your child's outer ear; do not use soap or allow water to enter the ear canal. If cotton is used to absorb drainage, replace it as soon as it becomes moist.
- **Protect the middle ear from exposure to water.** After insertion of tubes, many doctors recommend using earplugs while swimming during the months that the tubes are in place in order to prevent water (and potential bacteria) from entering the middle ear. However, several recent studies show that this precau-

tion is not necessary. You can discuss the issue with your doctor if you have concerns about water exposure. But whether or not your child is wearing earplugs, you should not allow her to dive into the water or swim deeper than five or six feet below the surface, as it is felt that the increased water pressure may allow water to enter the tubes; you should also avoid letting soapy water enter the ear, as soapy water appears to enter the ear tubes more easily than clear water.

- **Monitor for potential problems.** If your child develops pain in her ears, has drainage from the ear, or has difficulty hearing, you should call your doctor, describe the problem to her, and schedule a visit for your child to be evaluated.

Your ENT doctor may see your child in one month's time. If otorrhea (discharge from the ear) is present, it could be a sign of a new ear infection. The doctor will also assess the tubes and make sure that they are open and unobstructed (patent).

Often, the doctor will evaluate your child in six months and may assess hearing to make sure that her hearing improvements are sustained. She will check whether there has been a decrease in the number of ear infections since the surgery; most children experience a significant decrease in subsequent infections. She will also make sure that the tubes are still in place and functioning properly.

## What Are the Possible Complications of Tympanostomy Tube Insertion?

The most common problem after tympanostomy tube insertion is drainage from the ear, but there are a few other possible complications, which occur much less frequently.

### Blocked Tubes

The tubes can become temporarily blocked by excess secretions of mucus, particularly if your child has a cold or has any allergic conditions. To unblock the tubes, the doctor may prescribe special ear drops that you can apply to your child's ears for one to two weeks to help get the tubes functioning normally. It may not be possible to clear the tubes, but even so the doctor will most likely leave the blocked tubes in place, unless your child is experiencing ear pain or frequent ear infections. Allowing the tubes to come out on their own (rather than having to surgically remove them) promotes better healing of the eardrum.

### Tubes That Fall Out Early

The tubes usually stay in place for at least six to twelve months, helping your child through one winter season. However, in a few cases, tubes may fall out (extrude) early. Early extrusion could signal a technical problem with the way the tubes were inserted or that the design of the tube was not compatible with your child's ear, or that an active infection caused the tube to dislodge prematurely. The doctor will evaluate your child at this time and decide whether to try the surgery one more time using a different tube or to postpone the surgery until the next winter season.

### Tubes That Fail to Fall Out

In a few children, the tubes may stay in place longer than expected. If your child is not experiencing any problems with the tubes, the doctor will leave them in place for up to two or three years. After that point there is more risk of having a permanent perforation or hole in the eardrum (see below), and the doctor will remove the tubes surgically.

### Perforation That Fails to Heal

For the vast majority of children, after the tubes fall out, the hole in the eardrum closes back up on its own, but in a small percentage of cases, the perforation does not heal. Usually, the hole is small and does not cause any problems for a child; hearing is usually not affected. When a hole persists, most often a doctor will wait until a child is nine years old to surgically close the hole in a common and safe procedure called tympanoplasty. On rare occasions, if a child is having recurrent ear infections or hearing difficulties, then tympanoplasty would be considered at a younger age.

### Scarring of the Eardrum

In a small number of cases, when the perforation in the eardrum heals, whitish plaque forms, hardening the eardrum (tympanosclerosis). The scarring is usually mild and does not affect hearing. Scarring can occur from frequent or prolonged ear infections as well, but it is more common in children with tubes.

### Reaction to General Anesthesia

There is a risk of reaction to the anesthesia (generally characterized by dysfunction of the circulatory or respiratory systems). However, it is estimated that this occurs in less than 1 out of every 10,000 cases.

## What Are the Benefits and Limitations of Tympanostomy Tubes?

### Benefits

Insertion of tympanostomy tubes provides immediate relief of symptoms for most children. Excess fluid can drain from the middle ear, relieving pressure on the eardrum, and hearing is usually greatly improved. Tympanostomy tubes also provide long-term aeration of the middle ear, which promotes improved eustachian tube function and can help to prevent future infections. If your child does happen to get a subsequent ear infection, you will be able to tell immediately because you will see fluid draining from her ear. In addition, the infection will be easier to treat by using topical antibiotics, applied directly into the ear canal (see Chapter 4) rather than relying on oral antibiotics.

Many parents report that their children seem happier and more attentive because their ear discomfort is relieved and their hearing is improved. Some parents also find improvements in their children's balance, speech, and language abilities in the year following the surgery. Findings from surveys suggest that the majority of parents are pleased with the results of the surgery for their children.

### Limitations

Tympanostomy tubes are only effective during the time they stay in place. Your child may continue to have recurrent infections after the tubes come out; however, 80 percent of children require tubes to be inserted only one time.

In addition, tubes do not necessarily *prevent* future ear infections. While the majority of children experience *fewer* ear infections after surgery, some children with tubes still get one or two infections during a winter season.

# Adenoidectomy

Adenoidectomy involves surgical removal of the adenoids—tissue located in the throat near the back of the nasal cavity; an incision is made in the tissue and the mass of tissue is cut away. Removing chronically infected adenoids or enlarged adenoids that obstruct the eustachian tube and the nasal air passageway helps reduce risks for ear infections. Adenoidectomy is one of the most common surgical procedures performed on children in the United States; it is often performed to correct nasal obstruction and snoring and only selectively to treat ear infections.

## When Is Adenoidectomy Considered?

In general, adenoidectomy is considered for children over three years old with recurrent ear infections *and* signs of adenoid infection or enlargement. The ENT doctor will examine your child's palate, tonsils, throat, and nasal airways. She may evaluate the condition of the adenoids using several different techniques and ask you about any signs you may have noticed in your child, such as mouth breathing, snoring, or disturbances in her sleep. She will also review your child's history of ear infections and her response to previous treatments. The doctor will recommend adenoidectomy if your child has one of the following types of ear infections *coupled with* signs of enlarged adenoids or chronic adenoid infection (see below).

### Ear Infection History

- Recurrent AOM (more than three episodes in six months or more than four episodes in one year) that has not responded to antibiotic treatment or insertion of tympanostomy tubes

- Severe, incapacitating AOM characterized by intense ear pain, high fever, increasing hearing loss, or vertigo (feeling of dizziness) that has not responded to antibiotic treatment or insertion of tympanostomy tubes
- Chronic OME (fluid lasting longer than four to six months) when there are signs of hearing impairment, and that has not responded to antibiotic treatment or insertion of tympanostomy tubes
- Cases of repeat infections that occur after a child has already had tympanostomy tube insertion

### Enlarged Adenoids
- Enlarged (hypertrophied) adenoids causing obstruction of the nasal airway, impaired swallowing, mouth breathing, snoring, or sleep disturbances.

### Chronic Adenoid Infection
- Persisting nasal symptoms (such as runny nose or nasal congestion) of inflamed adenoids due to infection, after two courses of antibiotic therapy have been tried and failed; at least one of the courses should be with an antibiotic that is effective against resistant bacteria.

## Discussing Adenoidectomy with Your Doctor

If your ENT doctor is recommending adenoidectomy for your child, ask her to explain her reasons. If the doctor has found signs of infected or enlarged adenoids in your child and the ear infections are affecting her hearing or behavior, then adenoidectomy is a reasonable choice if your child is three years of age or older.

However, there are some situations where adenoidectomy might not be warranted:

- If your child is younger than three years of age

- If your child has not previously had ear tube surgery

- If your child is not showing signs of enlarged or infected adenoids

- If your child's ear infections are not causing hearing problems or speech and language delays

- If your child's ear infections are few in number and are responding to antibiotic treatment

By talking things over carefully with your doctor, together you can decide if adenoidectomy is the best choice for your child.

## How Is Adenoidectomy Performed?

Adenoidectomy is performed in a hospital under general anesthesia. The surgery is never done while a child still has an acute infection, only after the infection has subsided. Since bleeding is one of the uncommon but possible risks, it is important not to give your child aspirin or ibuprofen (Motrin, Advil) for two weeks before surgery. These medications may affect the ability of the blood to clot and increase the risk of intraoperative or postoperative bleeding.

On the day of the surgery, you will need to arrive at the hospital two to three hours before the scheduled operation. Your child will not be allowed to eat or drink anything for eight hours prior to the surgery in order to have the safest anesthesia experience possible. To help occupy your child during the wait, you can bring along a favorite toy or book. It is important to review some of the follow-up care that will be needed in the first week after the surgery. Feel free to ask questions if you do not fully understand something.

The anesthesiologist will meet with you to explain how the anesthesia will be administered (usually by breathing gas through a mask, which is followed by placement of a breathing tube). In addition, the ENT doctor who will be performing the surgery will stop by to talk with you briefly to see if you have any last-minute questions. When it is time for the procedure, you can accompany your child as far as the waiting area outside of the operating room.

Adenoidectomy generally takes about twenty to thirty minutes. The anesthesia is administered, incisions are made in the tissue, the adenoids are separated from the lining of the throat and removed. Different techniques are used to control bleeding in the mouth, such as applying pressure and use of a special electric coagulation device.

After the procedure your child will be brought to a recovery room, where you can rejoin her. Every child awakens from anesthesia differently. She may be a little groggy from the anesthesia. A nurse will prop your child's head up slightly, keeping it at a 45-degree angle to allow excess fluid to drain from her mouth; the nurse may also use suction to gently remove blood and mucus from her nose or mouth. Your child's throat may be sore. Swallowing will also be a little painful at first. The nurse will encourage your child to swallow normally and have sips of water; your child can try other fluids and then a little solid food after two hours.

During the hours after the surgery, your child will be monitored in several key areas:

- Airway. The nurse will suction off fluids from your child's nose and mouth in order to keep her airways clear and promote healing at the site of the incisions

- **Fluid intake.** Initially an intravenous line (IV) will be hooked up to a vein in your child's arm to maintain adequate fluids. Once your child is able to drink more liquids, the nurse can remove the IV.
- **Discomfort.** Your child will have mild pain after the surgery; she will feel some general discomfort from her sore throat and the effects of anesthesia. The nurse can give your child mild analgesic medications (nonaspirin pain relievers) to ease her discomfort. Encouraging your child to swallow sips of water also helps reduce soreness in the throat. Some children are irritable when they awaken from anesthesia.
- **Signs of infection.** Many children have a low-grade fever after the surgery that goes down in a few days. High fever is uncommon and could signal possible infection.
- **Excessive bleeding.** It is normal for small amounts of blood to drain from your child's mouth or nose in the hours following the surgery. Bleeding is rare, but if it occurs your child may need additional treatment.

You can provide comfort to your child by sitting with her, reading to her, or letting her listen to music or stories through headphones, activities that do not require her to talk. When your child meets the criteria needed for discharge, you will be able to take her home.

## What Is the Follow-up to Adenoidectomy?

The hospital staff should give you written information about follow-up care and discuss it with you to see whether you have any questions. There are some general precautions, such as mild restriction of physical activity. It may also help to keep your child away from anyone who might have a respiratory infection. There are several things you can do to help care for your child and speed recovery:

- **Ease ear and throat pain.** For the next few days after the surgery, your child may feel some pain in both her throat and ears. You can give your child a nonaspirin pain reliever as directed by your doctor to ease discomfort.
- **Encourage swallowing.** Swallowing may be mildly painful for a short period of time. Although your child will probably not feel like drinking much, you should encourage her to have plenty of liquids, as this will speed recovery. In addition, give your child only soft foods—nothing spicy or rough textured—to avoid irritating the throat.
- **Protect the incisions from infection.** It is important to clean your child's teeth regularly in the weeks after the surgery.
- **Treat possible constipation.** Your child's stools may be a bit black and tarry for a few days afterwards, due to blood swallowed during the operation. Many children also experience mild constipation. To relieve the constipation, encourage your child to drink juices and eat fruit.
- **Monitor for bleeding from the mouth or nose.** As the incisions heal, white scabs form over the site of the adenoids. If the scabs come off, bleeding may occur, usually seven to ten days after the surgery. If the bleeding does not stop, call the doctor; cases of excessive bleeding are very rare. In unusual cases of prolonged bleeding, you should bring your child back to the hospital for treatment.

Often, your ENT doctor will schedule a follow-up visit for two to four weeks after the surgery. For most children, vocal quality, breathing, and swallowing are all improved after an adenoidectomy.

The doctor may want to see your child again in one to six months to make sure that improvements in breathing and swallowing have been sustained. She will also want to find out whether your child has had fewer nasal or ear infections since the surgery. Most children experience a reduction in infections and less nasal obstruction, a key indicator that the surgery was effective.

## What Are the Possible Complications of Adenoidectomy?

Serious complications following adenoidectomy are rare, but it is important to be informed of the potential risks before giving your consent for the procedure.

### Immediate Postoperative Bleeding

Uncontrolled bleeding during the operation happens very rarely. If bleeding occurs and is not short-lived, your child should return to the hospital for evaluation and treatment.

### Delayed Bleeding

There is a small percentage of cases where bleeding from the nose or mouth occurs seven to ten days after the surgery. This can occur even when the surgery has gone smoothly. Prolonged bleeding will require treatment, and your child should return to the doctor for evaluation.

### Infection

There is a slight risk of infection at the site of the incision, but infection occurs infrequently and can be treated with antibiotics.

*Reaction to Anesthesia*

There are isolated cases of children having difficulty with anesthesia (generally characterized by dysfunction of the circulatory or respiratory systems). Anesthetic complications are very rare, occurring in less than 1 out of every 10,000 cases.

*Change in Vocal Quality*

A change in the quality (sound) of your child's voice is another possible complication seen after adenoidectomy. This change is usually temporary, but if the change in vocal quality persists, there are corrective measures that can be undertaken, such as speech therapy or additional surgery of the palate.

## What Are the Benefits and Limitations of Adenoidectomy?

*Benefits*

Most children who have had an adenoidectomy get fewer ear infections and experience improvements in breathing, vocal quality, and sleep (if enlarged adenoids were causing snoring or other sleep disturbances). Research suggests that these benefits are most pronounced in children who have had chronic otitis media with effusion (OME).

*Limitations*

A recent study on the *long-term* effects of adenoidectomy found that postoperative improvements in children's conditions are most significant during the first year following the surgery.

# Tonsillectomy

Tonsillectomy (removal of the tonsils) is no longer recommended as a primary treatment for ear infections. Research findings indicate that the procedure is not effective in improving middle ear function or preventing ear infections. In addition, research on the effects of tonsillectomy combined with adenoidectomy to treat ear infections found increased complications such as postoperative bleeding and dehydration and no significant decrease in the occurrence of ear infections.

## New Surgical Treatment: Laser-Assisted Myringotomy

A new laser surgery technique has recently been used by a few doctors to treat ear infections. In laser-assisted myringotomy (LAM), the doctor uses a laser to make a tiny hole in the eardrum to drain excess fluid from the ear and aerate the middle ear. The hole stays open longer than one made with a scalpel in the traditional myringotomy procedure (see page 108), remaining open typically two to four weeks as opposed to only three days. In addition, LAM has been tested for the insertion of tympanostomy tubes. An advantage of LAM over traditional ear tube surgery is that general anesthesia is not required and LAM can be done in a doctor's office. The indications for performing the LAM procedure have not been fully documented and are preliminary.

Research on the potential benefits and risks of LAM is also very limited. One study examined the long-term effect of LAM on 162 patients, and found that three quarters of them were considered cured. In contrast the success record with insertion of tympanostomy tubes is thought to be close to 90 percent. More research is needed to determine the effectiveness of LAM compared with that of traditional surgeries.

# Six

# Complementary and Alternative Treatments

Complementary and alternative medicine (also called CAM or alternative therapies) refers to a wide range of treatments that can include everything from acupuncture to herbal and homeopathic medicines. Other terms sometimes used for these types of therapy include natural, holistic, and integrative.

Many of the alternative therapies are based on a *holistic* approach (dealing with the body as a whole rather than segmented parts) to treating illness. Conventional (or traditional) medicine is based on the principle that disease occurs when an environmental agent overwhelms the body; to treat the illness, the infection must be fought with another environmental agent (such as antibiotics).

Over the past ten years, there has been a great increase in the use of alternative therapies in the United States to treat everything from colds to depression and memory loss. Surveys found that in 1997 people paid 629 million visits, with "out-of-pocket" expenditures of $21.2 billion, to see alternative practitioners. In addition, people spent $15 billion on alternative medicines (that is, herbal remedies and homeopathic medicines). However, findings also suggest that in most cases these therapies were used as a complement to, rather than a replacement for, conventional medical treatments. Some of the biggest increases have been in the use of herbal remedies, homeopathic medicines, and chiropractic, many of which are being used in some capacity to treat ear infections.

The key controversy surrounding use of alternative therapies is that very few have been proven effective in clinical trials (tests) for treating specific conditions (in comparison, many studies have been conducted on traditional pharmaceutical medications, although only a few medical procedures that are being performed on a daily basis have been well studied). The best way to test the effectiveness of a treatment is through a *randomized controlled trial.* In randomized controlled trials, people with similar conditions are randomly assigned to two or more treatment categories:

- The treatment to be studied (in this case, an alternative treatment)

- A conventional treatment (medical or surgical) termed "usual care" (the control group)

- No treatment, or a placebo (a "nonactive" treatment)

This method of study is the only way to assess whether an alternative treatment is more effective than conventional treatment or no treatment, an important point when treating ear infections, since the majority of infections resolve on their own. For example, a research study that has no randomization of its subjects and has no control group to compare the treatment being studied, and has a positive result cannot be trusted. A study of this design would fail to demonstrate efficacy, or effectiveness, of the selected treatment.

Although there have been numerous studies of several selected alternative therapies, the quality of the majority of research varies quite widely. There is no systematic collection of data for alternative practices, many of the methods used for measuring their effectiveness are flawed, and results of many studies are inconclusive. In addition, the findings of many studies have not been published or put up for review by other health care professionals (peer review), and only a small percentage of the research includes randomized controlled trials. The overall lack of scientific evidence on effectiveness is the primary reason that many members of the traditional medical community have objections to the use of alternative treatments. However, advocates for alternative practices point out that the effectiveness of many conventional procedures has also not been proven in scientific studies.

This variation in the quality of research has primarily been due to lack of interest by research institutions and lack of money for this research. This has subsequently changed over the past decade. Millions of dollars are now available through the federal government and are being spent to look at the effectiveness and efficacy of many alternative and complementary treatments for a wide range of medical conditions. With this increase in funding comes renewed interest from the academic community in making sense of this provocative and rapidly expanding field.

Because of the surge in use of alternative therapies by the public, the federal government is funding more investigations into the subject. In 1992, The National Institutes of Health (NIH, part of the U.S. Department of Health and Human Services) established the Office of Alternative Medicine. This office was established with an initial budget of $2 million. In 1998 through congressional mandate, this office was elevated to the status of a National Center— The National Center for Complementary and Alternative Medicines (NCCAM)—with a budget of $50 million. The budget has continued to grow and it is estimated that it will top 100 million dollars in 2001, making the NCCAM one of the fastest-growing centers at the NIH (although its funding is still a small part of the total NIH budget). The NCCAM is devoted to researching and disseminating information about alternative remedies; it has already produced publications on acupuncture and the herbal remedy for depression St. John's wort, and plans for further studies of alternative treatments are under way.

In 1998, the *Journal of the American Medical Association* devoted an entire issue to discussion of herbs and alternative remedies. Findings from one survey noted that many medical professionals use alternative therapies themselves. And even doctors who oppose use of alternative therapies agree that it is not enough to tell patients "they don't work, don't use them." There is general agreement that the medical community needs to become more informed about alternative therapies, and the majority of medical colleges now include courses in alternative and complementary medicine. Hopefully, the surge of new activities by health organizations and medical schools will build a greater scientific body of evidence regarding alternative treatments, providing health care professionals and consumers with new information.

In the meantime, what can you do as a parent if you are interested in trying an alternative treatment for your child's ear infection? First, discuss it with your doctor. Find out what he knows about alternative therapies, whether he is open to their use, and what type of therapies he might consider using. Second, do some research on your own as well (see Resources, page 227) to assess what types of therapies make sense for you and your child. Third, do not interrupt or stop a course of conventional treatment—if your child has already started one—in order to try an alternative therapy. However, if used selectively and with oversight from a health care professional, you may find that an alternative therapy is an appropriate complement to conventional treatment.

The following alternative treatments—herbal remedies, homeopathic medicines, and chiropractic—have been used in various ways to treat ear infections:

- To alleviate symptoms

- To counter the adverse effects of antibiotics

- To speed the recovery process

- To boost the immune system or overall health

As a parent, it is important for you to learn what is currently known about these therapies, including information about their effectiveness and safety, and precautions if using them for ear infections. While the information presented here is not comprehensive, it offers some preliminary guidance for sensible decision making regarding use of alternative therapies.

# Herbal Remedies

Herbal remedies contain plants or plant parts considered to have beneficial effects on tissues or organs. The active (beneficial) ingredient of a plant may be in the leaves, roots, fruit, flower, bark, stem, or seeds. Herbal remedies are available in many forms, including capsules and tablets, extracts or tinctures (herbs soaked in alcohol solution, although there are also alcohol-free extracts made specifically for children), and teas.

The notion of herbs as alternative medicine is somewhat misleading because many traditional prescription medications used today are derived from a plant source or contain chemical imitations of a plant compound. Aspirin is a chemical imitation of the substance salicin, found in the bark of the white willow tree. Ephedrine and pseudoephedrine, ingredients found in many cold remedies, are derived from the ephedra plant, which was used in China for centuries to treat colds and flu. Digitalis, derived from the foxglove plant, is used to treat heart conditions. However, these medications derived from plants have also undergone extensive research to test that they are safe and effective, a claim that cannot be made for most herbal remedies (see below).

## Effectiveness of Herbal Remedies

To date, the scientific evidence on the effectiveness of herbal remedies is limited. There has been no systematic collection of data on the use of herbs in the United States and there is inadequate assessment of many of the active chemical compounds found in herbs and how they act in the body during illness—or in good health. In addition, there is insufficient information on optimal preparation and dosages for many herbs. As a result herbal remedies are *not* recognized as medicines by the U.S. Food and Drug Administration (FDA).

The main body of research on medicinal herbs comes from studies in Europe and China; in Germany, where nearly 30 percent of medications prescribed are herbal and the production of herbal remedies is regulated by the government, over 200 herbs have been approved by the government for medical use; moreover, half of the prescriptions for herbal remedies come from doctors. Findings suggest that some herbs target specific organ systems in fighting illness, some act as a general tonic to promote overall health, and others help to soothe pain and inflammation. However, the studies vary greatly in quality and in providing evidence of effectiveness compared to other treatments. Even the *German Commission E Monographs: Therapeutic Guide to Herbal Medicines* notes that more research needs to be conducted on the use of herbal products. Unfortunately, there have been no published studies regarding the use of herbal remedies to treat ear infections.

Testing the effectiveness and safety of a product to receive approval for use in the United States can take years and cost millions of dollars. If a pharmaceutical company develops a medicine out of chemical imitations of plants or out of completely synthetic (nonplant) compounds and it is approved for use, the company is generally given exclusive rights (a patent) to market the product for a fairly lengthy time; the patent enables the company to recoup some of the money it has spent on research and testing. Herbs, on the other hand, cannot be patented, so there is little financial incentive for pharmaceutical companies to undertake extensive research on herbal remedies in the United States. Hopefully this picture will change over time as more research on herbs is conducted by the NIH and other health organizations.

## Safety and Risks of Herbal Remedies

Herbal products are not regulated in the United States as strictly as over-the-counter drugs or even foods—in contrast to some European countries where governments hold companies to strict standards for ingredients and manufacturing. Because the FDA considers herbal remedies as dietary supplements, not medicines, requirements are not as stringent regarding manufacturing and labeling of products. As a result, there is a lack of consistency among different manufacturers regarding the potency and form of the active chemical compound used in a remedy. Moreover, labeling can be misleading—some packages of herbal remedies do not indicate how much of an active ingredient is in each tablet or dosage and other ingredients may not be listed.

There has been no systematic collection of data on adverse effects of herbal remedies in the United States. One review of case reports found that during the past twenty years, nearly 100 fatalities and dozens of complications could be attributed to herbal remedies used in conjunction with pharmaceutical medications. The majority of reported complications were due to improper use of herbal remedies.

People tend to think herbs are harmless because they are "natural," but herbs are strong medicine and should not be overused or abused—just as with over-the-counter or prescription medications. High doses of herbs such as arnica, belladonna, and ephedra have been fatal. Other herbs such as arsenic are toxic in any quantity. Herbs may also cause allergic reactions in some people.

In addition, herbal remedies can interact with over-the-counter and prescription medications, although there is still inadequate information about such interactions. Even the recent *Physician's Desk Reference for Herbal Medicines,* which is published in the United States, does not include comprehensive information about possible hazards, contraindications (reasons for not taking an herbal remedy), and drug interactions. If your child has any medical conditions or is on prescription or over-the-counter medications, it is extremely important to consult with your pharmacist or doctor or another health care professional who is *knowledgeable* about drug-herb interactions and potentially dangerous side effects before considering use of any herbal remedy.

## Herbal Remedies Used to Treat Ear Infections

The herbs described below are considered helpful in fighting infections, particularly colds and flu. These herbal remedies are sometimes given for ear infections during and after a course of antibiotic therapy to help speed recovery and prevent recurrent infections, although it is important to remember that there is no conclusive evidence on the effectiveness of these herbs in treating ear infections. The herbs

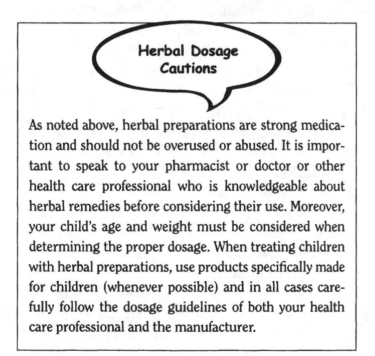

**Herbal Dosage Cautions**

As noted above, herbal preparations are strong medication and should not be overused or abused. It is important to speak to your pharmacist or doctor or other health care professional who is knowledgeable about herbal remedies before considering their use. Moreover, your child's age and weight must be considered when determining the proper dosage. When treating children with herbal preparations, use products specifically made for children (whenever possible) and in all cases carefully follow the dosage guidelines of both your health care professional and the manufacturer.

are listed by their commonly known name; the Latin botanical name, describing the family of plant it comes from, is listed in brackets.

### Echinacea (Echinacea angustifolia)

Echinacea is a pinkish coneflower plant grown in the United States. In laboratory tests, echinacea has been found to prevent the formation of an enzyme called hyaluronidase that destroys a natural barrier between healthy tissue and unwanted infectious agents. The herb is thought to help boost the immune system and fight against bacteria and viruses. European studies have found that echinacea can help to lessen the severity of colds and flu and help speed recovery. It is often taken when the first signs of cold or flu appear. Echinacea is considered safe for children with very little chance of any side effects. However, it should not be given on a daily basis for more than one to two weeks or it will lose its effectiveness.

### Goldenseal (Hydrastis canadensis)

Goldenseal is a plant that grows in the eastern United States. Its anti-inflammatory action helps to soothe irritated mucous membranes, and goldenseal is commonly used to relieve some of the symptoms of cold and flu. The herb is also thought to be effective against bacterial infection, but studies have not shown a specific protective mechanism. Goldenseal is a strong herb and it can raise blood pressure. It should be given in very small doses to children and should not be given on a daily basis for more than one to two weeks.

### Oregon Graperoot (Berberis aquifolium)

Oregon graperoot grows abundantly in the northwestern United States. It is considered an antibacterial herb; berberine is an antibioticlike chemical that helps stimulate the immune system. The herb is used for persistent illness (rather than as a preventive measure) to treat sinus infections and ear infections and is sometimes used as a substitute for goldenseal (see above).

### American Ginseng (Panax quinquefolius)

American ginseng is grown primarily in Wisconsin. It is thought to help the body cope better with stress and is commonly used following a bout of infection (and a course of antibiotics) to speed recovery and boost energy. The herb is a mild stimulant and should be used in very low doses with children. In addition, parents should be aware that there are two other types of ginseng that are not appropriate for children. Chinese ginseng (Panax ginseng) is a strong stimulant and can cause a jittery reaction. Siberian ginseng (Eleutherococcus senticosus) is used by athletes to increase stamina. It has also been found to help normalize blood pressure and lower blood cholesterol.

### Astragalus (Astragalus membranaceous)

Astragalus is grown primarily in China. Studies in Chinese medical journals suggest that astragalus helps activate the immune system, enhancing the body's natural ability to fight disease. It is commonly used for prevention, when the first signs of infection appear, or immediately following an illness to help speed recovery. Research also indicates that an extract from the plant may help to restore normal immune function in cancer patients with impaired immunity.

### Garlic (Allium sativum)

Biologist Louis Pasteur found garlic effective at killing bacteria in a lab experiment and garlic was used on the battlefield during both world wars to disinfect wounds and prevent gangrene. Garlic oil (from a capsule or in drops)—very lightly warmed and applied to the ear—is thought to relieve ear pain and help fight infection. Ear drops made with garlic, calendula, willow bark, and vitamin E are also thought to help support healthy functioning of the ear.

## Precautions if Using Herbal Remedies to Treat Ear Infections

If you are interested in trying an herbal remedy, first discuss it with your doctor at a well-child visit. Before buying any herbal remedies, you should be sure what the herb does, how to use it, and the possible side effects. If your child is currently taking over-the-counter or prescription medications, you also need information on potential herb-drug interactions. You can consult with your doctor, other health care professionals experienced with using herbs, or a reputable manual on herbs (see Resources, page 227). *Select reputable brand-name herbal remedies that have been made specifically for children and follow the recommended doses precisely.* Since there are no regulations in the United States concerning standardization in preparation of herbs, it is critical to look for a reputable company.

If your child is showing signs of a cold, an herbal remedy such as echinacea (alone or combined with goldenseal or Oregon graperoot) might be a reasonable alternative to over-the-counter medications to help treat the cold and prevent possible ear infection. Drops (taken orally) are usually the best form to use, dissolved in juice, tea, or broth. In general, it is better to give your child herbal remedies after eating since they may cause nausea if taken on an empty stomach.

If your child has symptoms of a potentially severe ear

infection—such as severe ear pain and a high fever—*do not* use herbal remedies. If the symptoms persist for more than twenty-four hours, call the doctor. Once the doctor has made a diagnosis and prescribed treatment, you can discuss with him whether any herbal remedies (such as astragalus or American ginseng) may be appropriate to help speed recovery during or after the treatment.

# Homeopathy

Homeopathy is based on the use of medications that are designed to stimulate the body's ability to heal itself. The practice of homeopathy dates to the turn of the nineteenth century, when a physician named Samuel Hahnemann began experimenting with some of the common medicines used at the time. He found that substances that would normally cause symptoms of illness in an otherwise healthy person could be used to treat ill persons with the same symptoms. With subsequent experiments he found that the smaller the dose of medication, the greater effect it had on the body's response system. The results of his experiments led to the development of a type of medicine that was gentle, preventive, and worked with the body's own system.

In homeopathic medicines, the active ingredient (usually a chemical compound derived from plants) is greatly diluted; a typical dilution is 1 to 1,000,000,000, meaning that there is 1 active part added to 999,999,999 parts water. In such dilutions, the active ingredient is not even present anymore, but the once present ingredient is thought to have an effect on the water molecules. (In homeopathy, the medicine is considered *more* potent at higher dilutions.) Research into homeopathic medicines is ongoing, but scientists have not been able to define a mechanism to explain how homeo-pathic medicines might work.

Traditionally, homeopathic medicines were prescribed by homeopaths—specialists in homeopathy. In the early 1900s several medical colleges included the study of homeopathy. The Hahnemann Medical College and Hospital, established in 1848 in Philadelphia, is still active today. Most home-opaths today are medical doctors, naturopaths (see Chapter 7), or some other licensed medical professional, and a few medical schools have begun including courses in homeopa-thy in their curriculum. Homeopaths traditionally tailor a remedy to the individual patient, based on the person's med-ical history and current health condition. A single or combi-nation medicine is tried at varying potencies to achieve the best effect; if after one month it fails to produce the desired result, a different homeopathic medicine or combination is tried.

## Effectiveness of Homeopathic Medicines

Many clinical studies (particularly in Europe, where use of homeopathic medicines is more widespread than in the United States) have found homeopathic medicines useful in treating a range of ailments including colds, hay fever, and migraine headaches, but the majority of studies have not compared effectiveness directly with the use of conventional medications. However, a few randomized controlled clinical trials found that homeopathic medicines were effective in treating both allergic asthma and diarrhea. There have been no randomized controlled trials of homeopathic medicines in the treatment of ear infections.

The medical community is divided on the issue of effec-tiveness of homeopathic drugs. Some health professionals believe in their use as a complement to conventional medications; others point out that many conventional treatments being used today have not undergone rigorous clinical testing either. Some health professionals suggest that homeopathy works because of the "placebo effect" (see below). Many health care providers feel that since the effectiveness of homeopathic medicines has not been proven conclusively through clinical studies, they have no place in the treatment of illness.

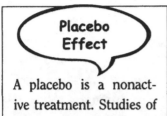

**Placebo Effect**

A placebo is a nonactive treatment. Studies of adults have found that some individuals respond to the placebo treatment simply because they believe they are getting medicine. This phenomenon is known as the placebo effect.

Because of the current rise in the use of homeopathic medicines by the general public, the NCCAM already has plans under way for clinical studies of homeopathic medicines. The findings should be useful in establishing the appropriate place for these drugs in treating illnesses.

In the meantime, the available information about use of homeopathic medicines to treat ear infections is very limited. Several homeopathic medicines have been used to relieve the symptoms, but there is no conclusive evidence of their ability to cure the infection.

## Safety of Homeopathic Medicines

Unlike herbal treatments, homeopathic medicines are well regulated. The *Homeopathic Pharmacopoeia of the United States (HPUS)*, established in 1897, is the official compendium of homeopathic drugs in this country and is recognized by the U.S. Food and Drug Administration as the official source of information and standards concerning homeopathic products. HPUS regulates the production and marketing of homeopathic drugs and ensures their safety and composition. In addition, homeopathic pharmaceutical manufacturers must follow strict production procedures and protocols set out in the FDA's *Compliance Policy Guide.*

Studies have found that homeopathic medicines are compatible with other medications and there have been very few reports of side effects. They are considered safe for infants and children if dosage guidelines are followed accurately. The main side effect that can occur is a condition called *proving,* in which an overdose of the active ingredient in the medicine produces the symptom that it is meant to cure. Proving happens only if a person continues to take a homeopathic medicine after the condition has cleared. The symptoms will usually end shortly after the person stops taking the medicine.

However, inappropriate use of homeopathic medicines carries risks. They are not suitable for acute conditions that require surgical intervention or immediate relief of symptoms. *The key danger for people using homeopathic medicines is the possibility of delaying the use of other effective conventional medical treatments to address acute or life-threatening conditions.*

## Homeopathic Medicines Used to Treat Ear Infections

The following medicines have been used to help alleviate a child's symptoms during ear infection; each one is geared to address specific symptoms. Some homeopathic products contain mixtures of three to eight substances, packaged as "combination remedies." (Some homeopaths believe that individual medicines, if appropriately chosen, work more effectively.) While there are individual reports by parents of success in using homeopathic medicines for ear infections, none of these medications have been proven in clinical trials to resolve ear infections.

- *Belladonna* to relieve severe, throbbing, ear pain and fever. (Caution: homeopathic medicines containing belladonna should not be confused with herbal remedies using belladonna; in undiluted form the herb is very strong and should not be given to children. However, the homeopathic form of belladonna is safe for children.)

- *Aconite* for sudden onset of ear pain, specifically following a cold

- *Ferrum phosphoricum* to treat fever connected with an earache

- *Hepar sulph* to treat earache with swollen glands

- *Kali muriacticum* to relieve nasal congestion and swollen glands

- *Pulsatilla* for moderate fever and gradual mild earache

- *Arnica* for children with tube placement, to help reduce inflammation surrounding the tube. (Caution: homeopathicmedicines containing arnica should not be confused with herbal remedies using arnica; in undiluted form the herb is very strong and should not be given to children. However, the homeopathic form of arnica is safe for children.)

## Precautions if Using Homeopathic Medicines to Treat Ear Infections

If you are interested in trying a homeopathic medicine to relieve your child's symptoms during an ear infection, you might want to discuss the matter in advance with your doctor at a well-child visit to find out his views on the use of homeopathic medicines. Some doctors are comfortable if you choose to see a homeopathic doctor as well. You should consult with a homeopathic doctor, pharmacist, or reputable guidebook (a list of resources is included in the back of this book) about which medications are appropriate for specific symptoms of ear infection and what potencies and dosages are correct for your child based on his age.

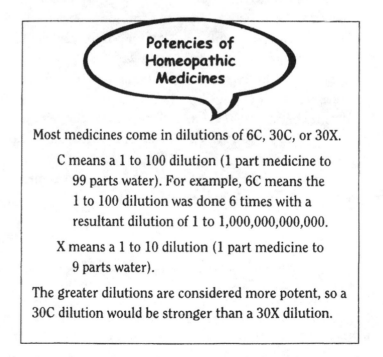

**Potencies of Homeopathic Medicines**

Most medicines come in dilutions of 6C, 30C, or 30X.

C means a 1 to 100 dilution (1 part medicine to 99 parts water). For example, 6C means the 1 to 100 dilution was done 6 times with a resultant dilution of 1 to 1,000,000,000,000.

X means a 1 to 10 dilution (1 part medicine to 9 parts water).

The greater dilutions are considered more potent, so a 30C dilution would be stronger than a 30X dilution.

In addition, you should be aware of some general guidelines in giving homeopathic medicines to your child:

- You can give the medicine more frequently if the symptoms are more severe, but do not exceed the recommended dosage for your child.

- Stop giving the medicine when the symptoms improve, a sign that the body is responding.

- Stop the remedy if there is no reaction after about six doses or if the symptoms change.

If you choose to use homeopathic medicines during the first few days that your child is experiencing symptoms of ear infection, make sure to select a medicine that is suited to your child's particular symptoms. Call your doctor after three days if the symptoms have not subsided. Once the doctor has confirmed a diagnosis of ear infection, you can discuss whether homeopathic medicines would be an appropriate complement to the suggested treatment options for your child's case.

If your child's symptoms are severe (strong ear pain, high fever) or are accompanied by a headache or a stiff neck, *do not* try homeopathic remedies—call your doctor immediately. These symptoms could indicate serious illness such as meningitis, which if left untreated can cause severe disability.

# Chiropractic and Massage

Chiropractic is a healing science that places emphasis on maintaining the structural integrity of the body. It is a method of health care delivery that places emphasis on the preventive aspects of health care. A chiropractor is not licensed to prescribe pharmaceutical medicines or perform surgery. The chiropractic philosophy states that aberrant (incorrect) motion or lack of motion of a joint will have a negative effect on the surrounding soft tissue (that is, the muscles and nerves) and will lead to interference with the transmission of nerve impulses in the nervous system; ultimately, this interference may result in dysfunction and disease. This loss of function in skeletal movement is treated using specific methods of spinal manipulation and massage. Treatment is noninvasive (does not involve surgery) and focuses on addressing the *cause* of the problem, rather than just palliating the symptoms. Chiropractic champions the need for early intervention through timely diagnosis and treatment.

Chiropractic principles are based on the premise that the nervous system has a central role in overall health and that body structure and mechanical function—particularly the condition of the spine—strongly affects the functioning of the nervous system. The bones of the spinal column (called vertebrae) interlink with muscles, ligaments, blood vessels, and nerves; the entire unit is known as the vertebral motor unit. When normal balance in this unit is disrupted—due to a loss or restriction of normal joint function (called a subluxation)—pain and dysfunction can result. For example, loss of full and complete joint motion in the neck (cervical spine) may interfere with nerve impulses to the brain and cause malfunctioning of one of the sense organs.

The first officially documented use of chiropractic in the United States took place in 1898, when Daniel David Palmer (who had learned about various bonesetting techniques used in other cultures) treated his first patient, Harvey Lillard, who had been complaining of backache and who was also hearing impaired. Not only was Lillard's back improved, but

## The Nervous System

The nervous system is one of the most complex of all the human body systems. More than 10 billion nerve cells are operating constantly all over the body to coordinate activities—both conscious and unconscious, voluntary and involuntary. Microscopic nerve cells, collected in bundles called nerves, carry electrical messages all over the body.

The *central nervous system* is composed of the brain and the spinal cord, a column of nervous tissue that runs through the bones of the spinal column.

The *peripheral nervous system* is made up of nerves from the brain (cranium) and spinal cord that branch out to connect to the rest of the body. Cranial nerves carry impulses between the brain and the head and neck. Spinal nerves carry messages between the spinal cord and the chest, abdomen, and arms and legs. The spinal and cranial nerves control muscle movements and also function in hearing and the other senses.

The *autonomic nervous system* is part of the peripheral system, and it controls involuntary (automatic) muscle movement, such as the pumping of the heart. This network of nerves carries impulses from the central nervous system to the glands, heart, blood vessels, and the involuntary muscles found in the walls of tubular-shaped organs such as the intestines, and hollow organs such as the stomach and bladder. Some of these nerves are *sympathetic,* meaning they stimulate the body in times of stress (increasing heart rate and blood pressure and also stimulating the production of adrenaline) and some of them are *parasympathetic.*

Parasympathetic nerves act as a balance for the sympathetic nerves, slowing down heart rate and lowering blood pressure.

### The Spinal Column

The spinal column is composed of twenty-six bone segments, called vertebrae, that are arranged in five divisions (see Figure 5). The first seven bones of the vertebral column, forming the neck bone, are the *cervical vertebrae,* starting at the base of the skull. There are twelve *thoracic vertebrae,* which link with the twelve pairs of ribs, and five *lumbar vertebrae* in the lower back. The *sacrum* is a slightly curved triangular-shaped bone below the lumber vertebrae. The *coccyx* or tailbone is the fused bone just below the sacrum. Between the vertebrae are discs made of cartilage, which help to provide flexibility and cushion shocks to the spinal column. The spinal cord (column of nerves) passes through the vertebrae of the spinal column.

his hearing (which he had lost suddenly seventeen years earlier after a "popping" had occurred in his spine) was restored.

Chiropractic treatment includes various forms of manual manipulation of the spine and peripheral joints (knees, elbows, etc.), massage, and exercises to increase mobility. Many chiropractors also counsel on nutrition and lifestyle changes. A typical visit includes taking a history of the patient's medical problems, a physical exam (similar to a conventional medical exam, including checking the pulse,

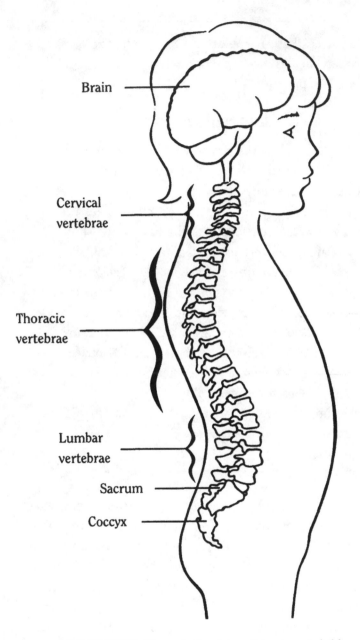

Brain

Cervical
vertebrae

Thoracic
vertebrae

Lumbar
vertebrae

Sacrum

Coccyx

FIGURE FIVE  The spinal column in a young child

154

blood pressure, and temperature) along with a functional exam to assess the mobility of the joints and flexibility, strength, conditioning, and tone of muscles.

When assessing mobility, the chiropractor uses a passive as well as an active movement of a joint within its normal range (this technique is called *mobilization*). Manipulation involves passive joint movement *beyond* the normal active range of movement. You can hear the joint "pop" as it is manipulated. There are over 100 distinct manipulation techniques with great variations in strength and speed; some movements are quick and strong, others are slow and gentle.

## Effectiveness of Chiropractic

Studies looking at the effects of spinal manipulation have found that it causes release of entrapped synovial fluid (fluid that nourishes and lubricates joints) and vertebral discs, reducing pain and restoring mobility to a joint. The full mechanism of how chiropractic works is still unknown and further studies are needed to fully understand it. The Foundation for Chiropractic Education and Research (FCER) is sponsoring further research in this area, and the federal government (NIH) recently funded grants to four chiropractic colleges to conduct biomechanical and anatomic studies.

Most people go to see a chiropractor because of back problems, and several studies in the United States have shown that chiropractic helps reduce lower back pain in adults, although not necessarily always restoring mobility as well. Studies in Britain, Canada, and Holland have also shown a positive impact of chiropractic treatment on the lower spine. However, the majority of research findings have had mixed results, and further studies are needed to provide more conclusive evidence. It should be noted that conventional medical and surgical treatments of lower back pain have had similarly inconclusive results in studies of their effectiveness.

Chiropractic has also been used to treat a range of other ailments, including dysmenorrhea (painful menstruation), colic, migraines, irritable bowel syndrome, and asthma. While there are individual reports of success in treating these problems, large-scale clinical studies are lacking. However, new findings are emerging from recent studies on the impact of chiropractic on internal organs. One study at the National College of Chiropractic found that certain techniques of manipulation on the thoracic spine increased activity in immune cells.

There is little information regarding the effectiveness of chiropractic for treatment of ear infections. Individual case reports suggest that spinal manipulation can be beneficial for relieving symptoms of otitis media with effusion (OME). A few preliminary studies have found that chiropractic is effective in improving some cases of ear infections and in reducing overall recurrence rates of infection. But these were not randomized controlled trials (see page 133), meaning the researchers did not test chiropractic against other forms of conventional treatments. Harvard Medical School, along with Boston Medical Center, has plans to recruit subjects for a randomized controlled trial, and study results should provide a clearer indication of the usefulness of chiropractic in treating ear infections.

## Safety of Chiropractic

At the turn of the last century, chiropractic was not regulated and patients were at risk from treatment by unqualified practitioners. Over the past twenty years, such risks no longer exist. The Council on Chiropractic Education (CCE) sets education standards and admission processes for chiropractic colleges in the United States and all operating colleges are fully accredited. All licensed chiropractors are also board certified by the National Board of Chiropractic Examiners.

There has been no systematic reporting of risks and complications associated with chiropractic. At the present time, most information comes from individual case reports and clinical trials. One study in Norway reviewed case reports of 1,058 patients and found that roughly half had experienced some side effects from the treatment (an average of four to five sessions). The main side effect was local discomfort in the area that was manipulated. A small portion of patients reported tiredness and headaches after the treatment. However, most of these effects were felt within four hours after the treatment and were not long-lasting. In addition, there were no serious complications noted. A review of case reports in the United States also indicates that serious complications are extremely rare.

## Chiropractic Techniques Used to Treat Ear Infections

Remember that a possible cause of ear infections is a blocked eustachian tube. The tube can become blocked if the muscle that opens and closes the tube (called the tensor veli palatini) is malfunctioning. The nerves that control the action of this muscle are part of a collection of nerves that extend through the first to fourth vertebrae of the neck (the cervical spine). In theory, any slight displacements in the first four vertebrae may affect nerve impulses in the pathways to the ear and cause malfunction of the tensor veli palatini, which may affect the opening of the eustachian tube. As a result the middle ear may not receive adequate ventilation, the eustachian tube becomes blocked, and fluid accumulates in the middle ear.

Theoretically, chiropractic treatment may be beneficial for OME by improving the functioning of the eustachian tube through manipulation of the upper spine (specifically of the first four cervical vertebrae in the neck) along with massage or "milking" of nearby lymph nodes. Manipulation is intended to release pressure on the nerves, remove interferences in nerve pathways, and improve function of the tensor veli palatini, allowing increased ventilation in the middle ear. The massage is performed to help the lymph nodes drain. This combined treatment may directly or indirectly influence the functioning of the eustachian tube, thus allowing for better drainage of accumulated fluids as well as help the tube ventilate the middle ear. The number of treatments varies, but four to five are the average. While some children do not respond to this treatment, other parents report great success. This type of anecdotal report is no substitute for randomized trials, however.

## Precautions if Using Chiropractic for Ear Infections

Your pediatrician or family physician is the most qualified to examine your child's ear to determine whether it is infected and what type of treatment is appropriate. If your doctor diagnoses OME, the standard recommendation is monitoring and observation for three months (at which time most cases resolve). If the fluid persists beyond three months, you may discuss with your doctor whether it is feasible to try chiropractic for one month (if hearing loss is not severe). Some parents may prefer an attempt at chiropractic before considering insertion of tympanostomy tubes (see

Chapter 5). Chiropractic is not recommended for children younger than three months of age.

If you choose to undertake sessions with a chiropractor, inquire of your doctor if he can suggest a chiropractor; if he has no experience with chiropractic referral, ask friends or relatives for a recommendation. If all else fails you can contact the American Chiropractic Association or International Chiropractic Association for a board-certified chiropractor in your area (see Resources). You may also want to continue to have your doctor monitor your child to see whether conditions change. If chiropractic treatment shows no results in one month (after six to eight treatments) you should consult again with your chiropractor before continuing further treatments; other treatment options may be more appropriate if your child is not responding to chiropractic. In addition, if your child's symptoms change, notify the doctor and chiropractor immediately.

If your medical doctor diagnoses acute suppurative otitis media (AOM) (characterized by accumulation of infected fluid in the middle ear), then chiropractic may not be advised. If your child has signs of ear pain, high fever, or swelling behind the ear, it could signal an acute infection or potential complication, which would require antibiotic therapy or surgery. The accepted guidelines that chiropractors follow instruct them to refer patients to a medical doctor if such acute conditions are suspected.

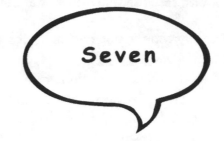

# Your Treatment Plan

Developing a plan for treating your child's ear infection is a joint effort between you, your doctor, and any other health care providers, such as specialists or alternative medicine practitioners, who may become involved in your child's care. Everyone has an important part to play in the process. As a parent you need to find out as much as possible about all of the available treatments—by both listening to your doctor's advice and doing some research on your own. You also need to think about your child's needs and consider what options you feel most comfortable with. Building a working relationship with your doctor in which you trust his advice but also feel free to voice your opinions is the best way to reach an agreement on the most appropriate treatment plan.

## Finding the Right Treatment for Your Child

Every case of ear infection is unique and your child's case needs to be assessed individually. A treatment that worked for your neighbor's child will not necessarily be appropriate for your child. You and your doctor will need to consider a range of factors, including your child's diagnosis, preexisting medical problems, treatment options, and possible risk factors. If the infections are recurrent, the potential underlying causes of the infection must also be considered. Deciding on an appropriate treatment will depend largely on how you answer the following key questions. (Refer to the Summary review of ear infections, page 162, as you read the following questions.)

## What Is the Diagnosis for Your Child?

Treatment options vary depending on what type of infection your child has and whether there is any hearing loss associated with the condition. If your doctor says simply that your child has an ear infection, ask him to explain what type of infection your child has and the reasons for his diagnosis.

## What Are the Treatment Options for the Particular Type of Infection Your Child Has?

There are usually several different treatment options for each type of infection; rarely is there only one correct treatment for an ear infection. Discuss all of the possible options with your doctor, assessing the risks and benefits of each one. Also take into consideration your child's history—for example, if there is any hearing loss or if his previous infections failed to respond to antibiotics.

In addition, remember that observation alone is usually an option, particularly if your child is not suffering from ear pain or a fever or if your child has some fluid in his ear but is experiencing no signs of hearing loss. Seventy to 80 percent of ear infections resolve on their own. As a parent, you can

## Ear Infections: A Summary Review

| Type of Infection | Characterized By |
| --- | --- |
| Acute suppurative otitis media (AOM) | Puslike fluid<br>Fever<br>Ear pain<br>Possible red or bulging eardrum |
| Otitis media with effusion (OME) (middle ear fluid) | Clear or mucuslike fluid<br>Possible hearing impairment<br>No fever<br>No pain |
| Recurrent AOM (3 or more episodes in a season) | Ear pain<br>Fever<br>Drainage from ear<br>Possible perforated eardrum<br>Possible hearing impairment |
| Chronic or recurrent OME (fluid persists for more than 3 months) | Blocked/plugged feeling in ear<br>Fluctuating hearing loss<br>No fever<br>No pain |
| Otitis externa (swimmer's ear; inflammation of the external ear canal) | Extreme pain<br>Inflamed, itchy skin in ear canal<br>Pus in ear canal, which may drain<br>Foul odor |

| Possible Causes | Conventional Treatment Options |
|---|---|
| Bacterial infection | Antibiotics |
| Viral infection | Allow 3–4 days for self-resolution (with medications to alleviate ear pain) |
| Eustachian tube obstruction | Monitoring and observation (allow 3 months for self-resolution) |
| Allergies | |
| Unresolved AOM | |
| Bacterial or viral infection | Antibiotics |
| | Address risk factors |
| | Adenoidectomy |
| Unresolved AOM | Antibiotics |
| Antibiotic-resistant bacteria | Address risk factors |
| Chronic adenoid infection | Address underlying causes |
| Partial immune deficiency | Tube surgery |
| Eustachian tube obstruction | Monitoring and observation (allow 4–6 months for self-resolution, as long as hearing loss in one ear is not greater than 20 dB) |
| Allergies | |
| Chronic adenoid infection | |
| Partial immune deficiency | |
| | Address risk factors |
| | Address underlying causes |
| | Tube surgery |
| | Adenoidectomy (if child is 3 years old or older and there are signs of adenoid infection) |
| Overexposure to water, leading to soft or to dry, cracked skin, allowing surface bacteria to break through skin barrier and cause inflammation | Cleaning of ear canal and ear drops |
| | To prevent future problems, earplugs and ear drops when swimming |

let your doctor know that you are open to simply monitoring your child's case, and together you can decide if observation is the best strategy for the time being.

### Is Your Child at Any Particular Risk for Ear Infections?

Even if it is your child's first case of ear infection, it is worthwhile to discuss with your doctor any factors that might make him more at risk for future infections, such as secondhand cigarette smoke or your day care setting (see Chapter 2). Your treatment plan could include preventive measures to minimize any risks for which you have some control (see Chapter 8).

### What Are the Potential Underlying Causes of Your Child's Infection?

If your child is having recurrent infections, you and your doctor may want to investigate possible underlying causes such as allergic conditions, adenoid infections or enlargement, or partial immune deficiencies before pursuing further treatment. If you are able to identify one or more potential causes, your treatment plan can include measures to address these conditions.

## Choosing a Health Care Provider

Your child's primary care doctor will be the central figure in treating your child's ear infections. Hopefully you are pleased with your doctor and you will have already established a good working relationship with him. In most cases, your doctor will be able to manage the care of your child's ear infections very well; pediatricians and family physicians generally have a great deal of experience handling ear infections, and have excellent rapport with children. Factors that may help you select your doctor include:

- If the doctor conducts an unhurried and thorough ear examination

- If the doctor explains fully and clearly the reasons for his diagnosis or for his recommended treatment

- If the doctor is open to discussing other possible treatment options

- If the doctor seems open to referring your child to a specialist

If you do not have a positive experience with your doctor and cannot improve the situation by talking to him or if you do not feel that your doctor understands or responds to your concerns, you may want to think about changing doctors. Finding a doctor whom you trust and with whom you feel comfortable will make coordinating your child's care much easier.

In certain situations, you and your primary care provider may want to consider referral to a medical specialist (an ear, nose, and throat, or ENT, doctor) or even alternative care provider (a naturopathic doctor, homeopath, or chiropractor). Bear in mind that in recent years, an increasing number of traditional medical schools are incorporating courses in spirituality and medicine, the mind-body connection, and alternative therapies into their curriculum, so more and more medical doctors are becoming familiar with this field.

Learning a little about each provider's training and background may help you to decide which additional health care provider may be appropriate for your child's care.

## Finding an ENT Doctor

ENT doctors (otolaryngologists) attend four years of undergraduate college or university followed by four years of medical college, then complete a one-year residency in surgery and a four- or five-year residency in illnesses of the ears, nose, sinuses, throat, and other structures in the head and neck. During their residency, the doctors spend time in clinics, hospitals, and operating rooms, building their patient skills. At the completion of their training, they take a comprehensive exam given by the American Board of Otolaryngology (a member board of the ABMS, see Resources), and can become Fellows of the American Academy of Otolaryngology—Head and Neck Surgery. Some ENT doctors complete additional years of study, learning about the ears, nose, and throat in a variety of fields, such as pediatrics, reconstructive surgery, head and neck cancers, or otology (ear problems). All ENT doctors are qualified to assess the need for surgical treatment of ear infections.

Your primary care doctor should give you referrals for at least two ENT doctors. You can also ask for recommendations from friends who have had a good experience with an ENT doctor in treating their child's ear infections. If possible, try to find an ENT doctor who has focused specifically on ear disorders in children. In addition, the American Academy of Otolaryngology—Head and Neck Surgery has a Web site that allows you to search for qualified doctors in your area (see Resources, page 228).

## Your Child's Primary Care Doctor

Primary care doctors, selected when (or before) a child is born, can include pediatricians and family physicians. Regardless of their specialty training, all medical doctors must pass a comprehensive licensing exam to be licensed by their state's medical board in order to practice medicine in their state.

Pediatricians are medical doctors who treat children and teenagers up until adulthood. Their training involves four years of college including premedical courses and four years of medical school, followed by a three-year pediatric residency with experience in hospitals and clinics. During their residency they work in several different departments, receiving a medical education covering various pediatric specialties. At the completion of their residency they may take a comprehensive exam given by the American Board of Pediatrics (a member board of the American Board of Medical Specialists, ABMS); pediatricians who pass this exam are "board certified" and can become Fellows (members) of the American Academy of Pediatrics (the initials FAAP may then appear after their name). Some pediatricians also take additional training for one to three years after their residency in a pediatric specialty such as pediatric cardiology (diagnosis and treatment of pediatric heart conditions).

Family physicians are medical doctors who treat all members of a family—children, teenagers, and adults—for a wide range of conditions. Their college and medical education is similar to that of pediatricians, but their residency occurs in a family practice center. They focus on six areas during their residency: internal medicine, pediatrics, obstetrics/gynecology, psychology and neurology, surgery, and community medicine. Following their residency, they take a comprehensive exam given by the American Board of Family Practice (a member board of the ABMS) and can become Fellows of the American Academy of Family Physicians (the initials FAAFP may then appear after their name).

It is always best to use a primary care provider who is board-certified in his specialty. You can easily check the board certification of your provider through the ABMS Web site (see Resources, page 231).

## Finding an Alternative Medicine Practitioner

If you are considering seeking an alternative medicine practitioner—also called complementary and alternative medicine (or CAM) practitioners, or providers—for care of your child's ear infections, discuss the matter with your primary doctor. If your doctor is strongly opposed to coordinating your child's care with an alternative practitioner, you may need to consider finding another doctor whose viewpoint is more in line with your own. In addition, you may need to check with your insurance company to see whether your health plan offers any coverage for such practitioners. Many plans offer coverage for a certain number of visits if the practitioner is a licensed professional (discussed below);

other plans do not include any type of coverage for such services.

You may be able to get a recommendation for an alternative practitioner from your doctor, if he happens to be knowledgeable about the subject. Moreover, if you have any friends whose children have had similar problems with ear infections, and who have had a positive experience with an alternative practitioner, they might be able to assist you with your search. There are also specific resources for information, depending upon the type of practitioner you choose (see Resources).

### Naturopathic Doctors

Qualified naturopathic doctors (NDs) attend four years of naturopathic medical college after completing at least three years of standard premedical college education (courses in chemistry, anatomy, and physiology). The first two years of naturopathic medical education focus on basic sciences and pathology (the study of diseases), similar to a traditional, or conventional, medical curriculum. The third and fourth years address the use of natural therapies including clinical nutrition, homeopathy, botanical medicine, hydrotherapy (the use of water, usually externally applied, to treat disease), physical medicine (the use of physical agents, such as heat, cold, and exercise, to treat disease), and counseling. Students also undergo about 1,000 hours of clinical training in which they work directly with patients in a clinic or other health care facility; naturopathic clinical training is not as extensive as that of medical doctors.

Naturopathic therapies are based on primary care and prevention and can also complement the treatments used by traditional, or conventional, medical doctors. Many NDs practice as primary health care providers and refer patients to appropriate medical specialists when needed.

In selecting a naturopathic doctor, you should make sure that he is licensed in the state in which he is working. Twelve states currently have licensing boards for naturopathic doctors (Alaska, Arizona, Connecticut, Hawaii, Maine, Montana, New Hampshire, Oregon, Utah, Vermont, and Washington). If your state does not have a licensing board, you need to verify that the practitioner successfully completed the courses at one of the three accredited naturopathic medical colleges (in Arizona, Oregon, and Washington); the accreditation process is still ongoing for a new program at a college in Connecticut. The Council on Naturopathic Medical Education (CNME) is the only agency recognized by the U.S. Department of Education to grant accreditation to colleges.

The issue of licensing and medical college attended is of particular importance in regard to NDs. Many "practicing" NDs have not completed programs at an accredited naturopathic medical college. These practitioners may be "certified" after completing correspondence programs, abbreviated courses, or monthly seminars. It is highly preferable to select a practitioner with the best credentials. The American Association of Naturopathic Physicians (AANP), based in McLean, Virginia, is the key organization that advocates for professional licensing, national standards of practice and care, peer review, and scientific research on naturopathic treatments; other naturopathic associations are opposed to any formal licensing or accreditation process. The AANP Web site offers a good initial resource for locating a reputable naturopathic doctor in your area (see the list of resources at the end of the book). If possible try to find an ND who specializes in working with children.

### Homeopaths

Homeopaths may be naturopathic doctors, medical doctors, chiropractors, acupuncturists, or other licensed health care professionals, such as a nurse. However, not all home-opaths are licensed medical professionals; training programs are open to unlicensed practitioners and laypeople as well who have completed course work in anatomy, physiology, and pathology (the study of diseases). Homeopathic training is also part of the curriculum of naturopathic schools (see above); however, not all naturopathic doctors specialize in homeopathy.

Homeopathic schools generally run three to four years, but courses meet only once or twice a month. Homeopathic education consists of instruction in the philosophy of home-opathic treatment, review of the various substances that comprise homeopathic medicines, and study of the texts and databases regarding the range of medications designed to treat specific symptoms. In addition, students learn how to take a person's case history (called case taking)—collecting extensive details about symptoms of acute and chronic con-ditions and the person's psychological state—and how to conduct case analysis (diagnosis of the conditions and identi-fication of appropriate homeopathic therapies). Many pro-grams do not offer clinical training, meaning that students do not receive direct hands-on experience working with patients; they may observe case taking at a clinic or by watching a videotaped case.

In selecting a homeopath, it is advisable to find one who is both a licensed medical professional (for example, a licensed medical or naturopathic doctor or chiropractor) and is certified by a leading homeopathy organization, such as the American Board of Homeotherapeutics, the Homeopathic Academy of Naturopathy Physicians, the Council on Homeopathic Certifi-cation, or the National Board of Homeopathic Examiners. In addition, it generally requires years of practical experience to fully understand the homeopathic systems of treatment.

If you are looking for a reputable homeopathic practitioner, the Homeopathic Academy of Naturopathic Physicians offers a database of practitioners, based on location (see Resources, page 230). In addition, you can check a local alternative health magazine or bulletin (often posted at health food stores) to find out if there are any ongoing homeopathic study groups in your area; study groups often know who the best homeopaths are in the area. In seeking information about the practitioner, try to find out whether he specializes in working with children and what experience he has dealing with ear infections, allergies, or other chronic conditions associated with ear infections.

### Chiropractor

Chiropractors attend a four-year program at a chiropractic college (after completing a minimum of four years undergraduate education including courses in biology, chemistry, physics, and psychology.) Chiropractic training consists of classes in the basic sciences (such as anatomy, physiology, pathology, biochemistry, and public health) and in the clinical sciences (such as radiology; obstetrics; pediatrics; and eye, ear, nose, and throat), and classes specific to chiropractic (such as chiropractic principles and practices and manipulative techniques). Following completion of the coursework there is a one-year clinical internship in an outpatient clinic affiliated with the chiropractic college. Some chiropractors continue with postgraduate education that includes a two- to three-year residency at chiropractic and medical facilities. They can then choose to specialize. Chiropractic specialties include pediatrics and family practice, orthopedics, radiology, sports medicine, rehabilitation, and neurology.

Following coursework and the clinical internship, chiropractors take a comprehensive exam given by the National Board of Chiropractic Examiners. Depending upon the state in which the chiropractor decides to practice, he must pass an additional comprehensive examination required by the state for licensure in that state. The title of Doctor of Chiropractic (DC) is awarded upon successful completion of coursework, internship, and the exams. There are eighteen chiropractic colleges in the United States and two in Canada. Accreditation for chiropractic programs and institutions is rendered by the Council on Chiropractic Education (CCE). There are state licensing boards in all fifty states and only graduates of accredited colleges are eligible to sit for licensing exams.

In selecting a chiropractor, you should seek a practitioner who specializes in pediatrics and who has experience treating ear infections. If you do not have a recommendation from your doctor, another health care provider, or a friend, the American Chiropractic Association or International Chiropractic Association (see Resources, page 227) offers a listing of practitioners by location.

## General Considerations

No matter what type of practitioner you choose, it makes sense to find a health care provider whom you trust, respect, and feel comfortable with. Besides the specific points discussed above there are some general considerations that can give you guidance as you meet with a new provider; choosing a doctor or other specialist is a personal and individual decision, so you may find that some of the points discussed are not as important to you. If you are not satisfied with the provider at an initial meeting, you can always decide to seek a second referral.

### Rapport with Children

Look for a health care provider who is patient and gentle with your child, talking to him, making him feel comfortable, even engaging his imagination. For example, during an ear examination using pneumatic otoscopy (blowing air into the ear canal to test the movement of the eardrum), one doctor may tell patients that he is looking for Big Bird in the child's ear to blow him a kiss. Many children respond well to such images and it keeps them calm and occupied during a visit to the doctor.

### Interaction with Parents

Look for a health care provider who encourages your participation in managing your child's care. For example, does the health care provider:

• Encourage your assistance in examinations when appropriate

• Allow you to ask questions

• Ask for your opinion

• Listen to your point of view

Finding a provider who is open to parental involvement can make it easier for you in trying to coordinate your child's care.

### Communication Skills

It is crucial to find a health care provider who communicates well and who will listen fully to you and then talk to you about your child's case. For example, during an ear exam, the ENT doctor should explain what he is doing, what he has seen, and what it means in terms of his diagnosis. Or if an alternative practitioner is recommending a treatment, he should explain the reasons for suggesting the treatment, and also discuss whether the therapies should be a complement to any conventional treatments.

A good communicator also tries to educate parents, providing them with useful information at initial and follow-up visits. For example, if you are taking your child to a chiropractor for the first time, the chiropractor may explain some of the basic principles of chiropractic and the kind of manipulations or massage techniques he uses to treat ear infections.

### Availability

The availability and accessibility of your health care provider are key concerns if you are caring for a child with recurrent ear infections. At your initial visit with a new provider, ask whether he or a nurse takes phone calls if you need to discuss new information or further details about your child's care. Some providers communicate with patients through e-mail. Whatever the method, it is important to feel that you can get in touch with your provider if you need to, especially in the case of an urgent situation or emergency.

### Solo vs. Group Practice

If your health care provider is in a group practice, you might not always be able to see the same person; on some occasions another member of the group practice would see your child. If you are not comfortable with such an arrangement, you should find out whether it is possible to request your provider specifically when scheduling visits, and also find out what his accessibility is in case of an emergency (see above).

# Coordinating Care Between Different Health Care Providers

## ENT Doctor

The ENT doctor should establish a good rapport with your primary doctor, sending a report to your doctor after the first consultation, and making recommendations for further treatment in consultation with your doctor. As a parent you want to make sure good lines of communication stay open between the specialist and your primary doctor if your child continues to see the specialist. Check that the ENT doctor reports back to your doctor after subsequent visits and consult with your doctor as well as with your specialist if you have questions or concerns about the specialist's recommendations.

## Alternative Medicine Practitioner

No matter what alternative medicine practitioner you choose, make sure that your primary doctor (and the ENT doctor if you have one) is aware of your decision. Your primary doctor should still continue to monitor your child's care, so you should arrange a schedule of follow-up visits after you have seen the alternative practitioner. In addition, your primary doctor should receive reports and recommendations from your alternative-medicine practitioner. Some doctors may be open to such communication; others may not wish to have any involvement with an alternative practitioner or vice versa. As the parent, you may want to reconsider your involvement with any practitioner, medical or otherwise, who is not willing to communicate with others in the care of your child.

# Being an Informed Consumer of Medical Services

Even if you have a primary doctor (and other health care providers) whom you trust and respect, it is important that you give your input on decisions concerning your child's care. The best way to offer input is to learn as much as you can about your child's condition and the various factors that affect decisions about treatment.

Reading books and articles and conducting research through the Internet on treatment and prevention strategies are good ways to gather information. If you are using the Internet, be discriminating about the sources you consult because not all information found on-line is reliable. In general it is a good idea to refer to Web sites of reputable health organizations, such as the American Association of Pediatrics, or government agencies, such as the National Institutes of Health. (A list of resources, including Web sites, is provided in the Resources section.) If you are interested in investigating use of alternative therapies, consult professional handbooks or compendiums regarding herbs and homeopathic medicines (see Resources). Such texts are more reliable than brief self-help guides you might find in a health food store.

You may feel a bit overwhelmed at first when researching topics, but try to focus on one or two specific issues that are of most concern to you in your child's case; this focus will guide you as you sift through the wealth of information available. Most likely your health care provider will respond positively when you can share relevant information in discussions about your child's care.

With your doctor's guidance, you can also learn how to help monitor your child's care:

- By learning the symptoms of ear infections, you can assess when it is necessary to take your child to the doctor.

- By recognizing signs of treatment failure, you will know when to notify the doctor and when to start discussing other treatment options.

- By becoming familiar with indicators of hearing problems or speech and language delays, you can provide more precise information to your doctor for making decisions about managing your child's care.

# Being an Advocate for Your Child

Having a sick child creates a stressful situation; you may be anxious, confused, or frustrated in the midst of trying to help your child feel better. It can be difficult to think clearly, ask questions, and make decisions. At such times, it is important to remind yourself that you know your child best, and that your job is to stand up for what you think is right for your child.

Even if you find it difficult to speak up during your visit to the doctor (or other health care provider), *do not remain silent*. Your visit is a crucial time to get information, ask questions, and build on your relationship with your child's doctor. Make sure that you understand your doctor's diagnosis and all of the treatment options. If you question your doctor's selection of treatment, talk to him about it, and take your time to consider other options. There are very few cases of ear infection that present an emergency situation that needs to be handled immediately.

If you feel constrained trying to talk to the doctor during a visit when his time is restricted or your child is crying, see if you can schedule a phone appointment with him at a later time to discuss your child's case more thoroughly. This will also give you time to reflect on everything the doctor has said. You can think about what other questions you have (write them down), and you can also seek further information on your own before speaking to the doctor again.

It is helpful to be interested but not adversarial in advocating for your child; you simply need to ask questions, voice your opinions, and make sure that decisions are made using all of the available information. If you think your child's ear infections are causing her problems with hearing, speech, or behavior, let your doctor know. If you think the cause of recurrence of infection in your child is due to something other than what the doctor suspects, trust your intuition and share your thoughts. Your intuition may not always be correct, but it might provide the doctor with more clues so that together you can determine the most probable cause of infections and the most appropriate treatment options. Remember, you and your doctor share the common goal of restoring your child to good health.

If you are seeing an ENT doctor and he recommends a treatment, such as surgery to insert tympanostomy tubes (see Chapter 5), you should feel free to ask for a second opinion if you have reservations. Some insurance companies may also require a second opinion to be rendered before granting approval to cover a surgical procedure. If you receive a conflicting second opinion, it is important for the second specialist to consult with you, your ENT doctor, and your primary doctor to determine the reasons for the differences of opinion and to decide how these differences can be resolved in selecting an appropriate treatment.

# Partnering with Your Health Care Providers

While your primary doctor is the main authority on your child's medical condition, you are an equal partner in care and you need to work together with the doctor (and any other health care providers involved, such as an ENT specialist or alternative practitioner) to achieve the optimum care for your child. Start by building a good working relationship with your doctor (and any other providers you may be seeing). Let him know that you want to take an active role in managing your child's case and that you want to participate in decisions.

Decide on mutual goals for managing your child's care; seek answers to causes of the infection and develop prevention and treatment strategies together. If you have differences of opinion, discuss them openly, and come to a reasonable agreement that satisfies all parties. If you are honest about your views and informed about your child's condition and possible treatment options, the doctor (and other health care providers) should respect your opinions and value your contribution. Likewise, if you have chosen a doctor in whom you have confidence, you can trust his judgment when you feel unsure of the best course of action to take.

There are several ways you can contribute to managing your child's care with your health care providers.

- Keep a diary of your child's history of ear infections: when the infections began, the diagnosis, the number of infections he had during a winter season, whether one ear was affected more than the other, and the medications that were tried.

- Monitor your child's current situation: note his responses to treatment (or to observation).

- Provide information to your doctor about possible risk factors or underlying causes of your child's ear infection (see Chapter 2).

- Ask questions about the diagnosis and the recommended treatment.

- Do research on your own about treatment and prevention strategies.

- Facilitate communication between your doctor and other health care providers.

- Be sure to comply with giving the full duration of any prescription medication—giving it the prescribed number of times each day for the correct number of days.

---

## A Personal Experience:
### Being a Partner in Your Child's Care

It was Carlo's first ear infection since the family had moved to a new city, but his mother, Maria, was prepared for their visit to the new pediatrician. She and her four-year-old son had already met the new doctor on a short introductory visit a few months earlier, and she had spoken to him a few times on the phone since then. Also, her son's last pediatrician had already transferred copies of Carlo's records to the new doctor.

Carlo had experienced five or six ear infections in the past two years, which included a variety of treatments. Maria had also kept her own diary of her son's infections. In it she commented on such things as symptoms, the duration of the infections, and the type of treatments that were given and whether they worked or not. She brought this diary with her for the doctor's visit, along with her observations of his current illness. Her personal notes along with the transferred medical records provided the new doctor with a good review of her son's past infections and treatments—information that proved invaluable when designing a treatment plan for his current illness.

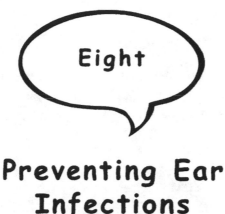

Eight

# Preventing Ear Infections

While your main concern is treating your child's ear infections when they occur, you also need to think about how to *prevent* future infections or at least reduce the risk of recurrent infections. Prevention strategies provide you a way to be proactive in caring for your child. In addition, such strategies may help promote your child's overall health and minimize her vulnerability to other infections as well.

The following suggestions offer basic guidance in preventing ear infections. However, not every point may be applicable or appropriate for your child's particular situation. In making decisions about prevention strategies, seek your doctor's advice, conduct research on your own, and take steps that make sense for you, your child, and your household. If you are unsure about using a particular preventive measure, the general "rule of thumb" is that if the measure has no harmful side effects, and there is a chance it might help in prevention, then it is worthwhile to undertake it as a precaution. Note that none of the suggestions presented in this chapter are known to have adverse effects.

# Maintaining Overall Good Health

To prevent ear infections, the best place to start is by promoting your child's overall good health. Hopefully you have already undertaken all of the following steps, but a brief reminder may still be helpful.

## Well-Care Visits

Just as it is necessary for mothers to see their obstetrician regularly during pregnancy to ensure a healthy fetus, it is equally important to take your child to the doctor regularly from birth onward. Well-care visits are an important time not only to check for signs of illness but also to monitor your child's growth and development—particularly during the first two years of life—to make sure she is progressing as expected. Well-care visits include assessment of hearing and basic speech and language development. Part of your well-care visits should include the standard schedule of vaccinations (immunizations) recommended for all children to protect them against serious childhood illnesses such as polio and the measles; see page 187 for a discussion of vaccinations and immunizations, including the new *Streptococcus pneumoniae* vaccine.

Well-care visits are also a crucial time for you to establish a productive working relationship with your child's doctor. As a parent, you can use the well-care visits to ask questions, get information, and express any concerns you may have about your child's health or behavior. Having positive experiences during these visits will also help during your special illness visits for ear infections.

## Nutrition

If your child is old enough to eat solid foods, try to offer her a well-rounded diet including fruits; vegetables; whole-grain breads, cereals, and pasta; and protein foods (such as meat, poultry, fish, and dairy products). Remember that certain vitamins and minerals play an important role in strengthening the immune system (see Chapter 2), so be particularly mindful of including foods in your child's diet that are rich in vitamin A, vitamin E, and zinc.

- Sources of vitamin A: yellow and orange squash, melons, green leafy vegetables

- Sources of vitamin E: vegetable oils, nuts, wheat germ, flaxseed

- Sources of zinc: fish, poultry, meat, legumes, dairy products

In addition, try to limit the amount of saturated fats and hydrogenated oils your child consumes since these types of fats are thought to have a negative effect on the body's anti-inflammatory mechanisms (see Chapter 2). However, in this era of fat-free foods, it is important to ensure that your child consumes enough fat—approximately 30 percent of her total calories should come from fat. Helping and teaching your child to make healthy food choices is an important way you can help her grow up to become a healthy adult.

Most children go through various stages when their eating habits may be problematic; they may not want to eat much or may only eat a few specific foods. Even if your child has days when she only eats peanut butter, crackers, and juice, do not be overly worried. Keep trying to offer her a variety of foods to encourage her to find healthy items that she does like. Most children tend to graze throughout the day rather than eat three large meals. It is natural for a child to eat only when hungry, and it is not wise to force your child to eat when she is not hungry.

Remember that most children are able to maintain a healthy diet based on the foods they eat. If your child does not have a healthy diet and you are concerned that your child is not getting adequate vitamins, minerals, or proteins, check with your doctor, alternative medicine provider, or pharmacist about using nutritional supplements (such as a multivitamin tablet or vitamin drops). You should purchase supplements based on the advice of your doctor, a nutritionist, or another health professional. In addition, there are a few general guidelines for selecting and using supplements for your child.

- Select a reputable brand-name product.

- Select supplements that are made specifically for children.

- Follow the recommended dosage.

- Choose supplements that are hypoallergenic.

- Avoid supplements with sugar and/or artificial flavors, colors, or preservatives.

- Select supplements that contain natural, not synthetic, forms of vitamins.

- Give your child supplements at mealtimes; they work together with the digestive process. Because they are concentrated, if taken on an empty stomach, they can cause stomach upset.

## Reducing Stressful Situations

Changes in your living situation such as a move, change of job, a new baby-sitter, or having a new child may create added stress for you, your spouse, and other members of your household. Young children often sense stressful behavior in their parents and may be affected by it as well. Stress can make it more difficult for the body to fight infection (which is why rest is so important when you are sick). If your child seems more vulnerable to infections, you may want to limit or restrict stressful changes, especially during the winter months or when your child is between six and twenty-four months old. If the change is unavoidable, you can take extra measures to compensate, such as spending extra time with your child, planning a special trip or event, or simply comforting and reassuring your child to help her adjust to the transition.

# Protecting Your Child Against Infections

Your child is more susceptible to illness during the first five years of her life, because her immune system has not yet fully developed, but there are measures you can take to protect your child from infections.

## Standard Vaccinations

Part of your well-care visits should include the standard schedule of vaccinations (immunizations) recommended for all children to protect them against serious childhood illnesses. Most of these vaccinations are given during the first

### Recommended Immunization Schedules for Children—January–December 2001

| Vaccine | How Often and Age Given | Alternative or Booster Age |
| --- | --- | --- |
| Hepatitis B | Given three times:<br>Birth–2 months<br>1–4 months<br>6–18 months | 11–12 years<br>(if previous<br>series was<br>missed) |
| Diphtheria, tetanus (lock-jaw), pertussis (whooping cough) (DtaP) | Given 5 times:<br>2 months<br>4 months<br>6 months<br>15–18 months<br>4–6 years | 11–12 years<br>(tetanus,<br>diphtheria,<br>only) |
| Hempohilus influenzae type B (Hib) | Given 4 times:<br>2 months<br>4 months<br>6 months<br>12–15 months | |
| Polio† | Given 4 times:<br>2 months<br>4 months<br>6–18 months<br>4–6 years | |

| Vaccine | How Often and Age Given | Alternative or Booster Age |
|---|---|---|
| Pneumococcal conjugate (Streptococcus pneumoniae [Prevnar] vaccine; (see also *Streptococcus pneumoniae* vaccine, below) | Given 4 times: 2 months 4 months 6 months 12–15 months | |
| Measles, Mumps, Rubella (MMR) | Given 2 times: 12–15 months 4–6 years | 11–12 years (if 2nd dose not previously given) |
| Varicella (chicken pox) | Given 1 time: 12–18 months | 11–12 years (if previous dose not given) |

\* Always consult with your doctor to see whether any adjustments are necessary in your child's immunizations, based on any medical conditions your child might have.

† Inactive polio vaccine (IPV) is recommended for all children in the United States rather than oral/live vaccine (OPV).

two years of a child's life. Recommended immunization schedules for children (see page 188) are published by the American Academy of Pediatrics in a report called *The Red Book*.

You should keep track of your child's immunizations to make sure she is up-to-date. In addition, if your child is too sick to receive her vaccination at a scheduled visit, make sure you reschedule the immunization once she has recovered. Your doctor should provide you with information about each of the vaccinations before your child is scheduled to receive them. You can also check with your doctor about updates on additional vaccinations (discussed later in this chapter). You can find further information on immunizations through the Web sites of the American Academy of Pediatrics and the Centers for Disease Control and Prevention (see Resources, page 229).

## Additional Vaccinations

In addition to the standard immunizations, there are other vaccines that protect against bacterial and viral infections and that offer new promise for parents in preventing ear infections. Many of these vaccinations are still in development, but you can ask your doctor for the latest information at a well-care visit, particularly if your child suffers from frequent respiratory illnesses in the winter.

### Vaccinations Against Bacterial Infections

Remember that three types of bacteria are thought to cause the majority of ear infections: *Streptococcus pneumoniae, Hempohilus influenzae, and Moraxella catarrhalis* (see Chapter 2). A new vaccine against *S. pneumoniae* (Prevnar) is now part of the standard immunization schedule, and vaccines are currently being developed to protect against the

**Streptococcus pneumoniae Vaccine**

Recently a vaccine (Prevnar) effective against seven strains of the *Streptococcus pneumoniae* bacteria (there are estimated to be ninety strains of the bacteria) was recommended for use in children as young as two months old; the vaccine can be given at the same time as other commonly recommended childhood vaccines. *S. pneumoniae* is believed to be a leading cause of ear infections.

Prevnar is well tolerated, with the most common side effect mild soreness and redness at the site of injection. The vaccine is increasingly important given the emergence of numerous antibiotic-resistant strains of *S. pneumoniae* (see Chapter 4), which is a leading cause of bacterial infections in young children. Prevnar is also recommended for older children (24 to 59 months) who are at particularly high risk of infection, such as children infected with HIV (the AIDS virus), children who have sickle cell anemia, and perhaps children who are considered "otitis prone." Children at high risk who are older than 24 months can also be given a different *S. pneumoniae* vaccine that will protect them against twenty-three strains of the bacteria.

strain of *Hempohilus influenzae* that is involved in ear infections and also to protect against *Moraxella catarrhalis*.

- *Hempohilus influenzae vaccine:* A vaccine against *H. influenzae type b* (Hib) is part of standard childhood immunizations, but type b is not found in ear infections. Developing a vaccine against the particular strain of *H. influenzae* that causes ear infections is difficult because it does not have the same structure that other types of *H. influenzae* have. Efforts are still under way to develop a vaccine that could offer protection against the strains that cause ear infections.

- *Moraxella catarrhalis:* Researchers are making progress on a vaccine to protect against *M. catarrhalis* as part of a project to develop a multiple vaccine that would be effective in fighting all three bacteria, particularly the strains that are resistant to antibiotics

### Vaccinations Against Viral Infections

Research is being conducted on the development of vaccines to protect against viruses that cause the respiratory infections linked to ear infections. Recently, researchers identified three types of viruses found in the middle ear of children with acute suppurative otitis media (AOM) (characterized by accumulation of infected fluid in the middle ear): respiratory syncytial virus (identified the most often), parainfluenza virus, and influenza virus.

More large-scale studies need to be conducted to confirm these findings, but researchers have concluded that a vaccine against respiratory syncytial virus may be a viable preventive measure against ear infections in the future. Development of a vaccine for RSV is a high priority as the virus is the most common cause of bronchiolitis and pneumonia (lung infections) in infants and young children.

Flu shots (influenzae vaccine), administered at the start of the winter season, may also have a protective effect against ear infections. In fact, a reduction in the rate of ear infections has been seen in studies of children who had received a flu shot, compared to other children who had not been given a shot. Reduced risk of flu minimizes the chances for viruses to cause swelling of the lining of the eustachian tube and eustachian tube dysfunction, which should therefore decrease the occurrence of ear infections.

## Restricting Exposure to Sources of Infection

Limiting your child's exposure to possible sources of infection, particularly during winter months, can help reduce the chances of acquiring viral and bacterial infections that lead to ear infections. These tips are particularly important when your child is in the crucial period of vulnerability for ear infections, between ages six and twenty-four months.

- Keep your child away from other children and adults who have colds, the flu, or other viral and bacterial infections.

- Avoid enclosed places with crowds of people such as movie theaters or airplanes.

- Wash your child's hands frequently, especially before eating.

- Wash your child's toys, pacifiers, and bedding frequently, especially after these objects come into contact with other children.

- Use disinfectant (*not* antibacterial) sprays in areas of your home such as doorknobs, the bathroom,

and kitchen where your child is most likely to
come into contact with germs.

## Inhibiting Growth of Bacteria in the Mouth

Preliminary research on gum containing xylitol sweet-
ener (a sugar made from wood) suggests that xylitol may
inhibit the growth of some bacteria in the mouth, including
*Streptococcus pneumoniae.* Xylitol gum is mainly used to
help prevent dental cavities, and two recent studies have also
shown that chewing xylitol gum can lower the occurrence of
ear infections in children. If your child is old enough to chew
gum, you may want to offer her xylitol gum—Xylichew is one
brand—after meals during the winter season, particularly if
she shows signs of a cold. It is not clear, however, how much
xylitol gum a child would need to chew for it to be most effective. Moreover, since gum chewing in general is not recommended for children younger than five years and most ear
infections are in young children, the benefits of chewing
xylotil gum will not be available for the children who are most
susceptible to ear infections. Xylitol chewing gum can be pur-
chased without a prescription, but you can speak to your dentist should you have any questions regarding its use.

Remember, in general, good oral hygiene—visits to the
dentist and brushing and flossing the teeth—is important to
control the growth of bacteria in the mouth and to prevent
dental cavities.

# Promoting Healthy Ears

There are a few simple measures you can use to maintain
healthy ears for your child. While these measures have not

been clinically proven to prevent middle ear infections, they are not harmful and may help to reduce risk of recurrent infection.

## Care Regarding Water in the Ears

Letting the ears get wet will not cause middle ear infections. So you should feel free to wash your child's ears during a bath and allow her to go swimming (if your child has ear tubes, see Chapter 5 for further information regarding water in the ears). However, it is important to dry your child's ears after a bath and particularly after swimming. If excess water remains in the ear for prolonged periods of time, the external ear canal can become soft and waterlogged, making it easier for bacteria to infect the ear canal of the outer ear, an infection known as otitis externa, or swimmer's ear (see Preventing Swimmer's Ear, below, and Chapter 1).

## Care Regarding Wax in the Ears

Wax in the ears does not promote ear infections; however, a buildup of excess wax can make it difficult for the doctor to examine your child's ears and can have an effect on hearing. To prevent buildup of wax you can wipe your child's outer ear periodically with a washcloth to remove the excess wax that reaches the outer surface from the ear canal. If the wax becomes hardened in the ear canal, consult your doctor regarding wax removal. Special ear drops are available to help soften the wax and wipe it away, but speak to your doctor first if you are thinking about using drops to prevent wax buildup. Do not put any cotton swabs in the ear canal; using cotton swabs can cause the ear to produce more wax, can pack the wax closer to the eardrum making the wax more

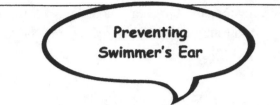

Infection of the outer ear (otitis externa, or swimmer's ear) is a common condition among certain children following water exposure, but can be prevented and easily treated. Swimmer's ear is unrelated to middle ear infections (otitis media) and does not lead to or cause middle ear infections, although at times its symptoms may resemble those of otitis media. You can take steps to prevent swimmer's ear by preventing the outer ear from becoming waterlogged:

- Pat dry the external ear and carefully dry the opening of the ear canal with a towel. If your child has water stuck in her ear, tilt her head to one side, have her shake her head gently, and pull the ear slightly in different directions to help the water drain out. Let the towel serve as a wick to remove any remaining water from the external ear canal.
- If your child is swimming frequently, you can check with your doctor about applying special ear drops to your child's ears before swimming. Some doctors recommend putting a few drops of rubbing alcohol—often mixed with a little vinegar, which inhibits the growth of bacteria on the skin—in the ears after they get wet to facilitate drying.
- Consider using earplugs and ear drops when swimming, to prevent water from entering the external ear canal; this may prevent future cases of swimmer's ear.

difficult to remove, and there is a risk of harming the eardrum if your child moves suddenly.

## Eustachian Tube Function

The eustachian tube (the passageway that connects the
middle ear to the nasal cavity and the throat) plays an important role in maintaining healthy ears because it allows excess
fluid to drain out of the middle ear and also ventilates the
middle ear cavity (see Chapter 1). The eustachian tube normally drains during swallowing, yawning, and crying. To
help promote drainage of fluids from the middle ear, you can
encourage your child to swallow frequently, especially when
she has a cold. The swallowing action is also thought to help
improve efficient opening and closing of the eustachian
tube. If your child is starting to get a cold, you can offer
young children drinks or a teething toy (if an infant) to
encourage more frequent swallowing.

In addition, if you are traveling by airplane, give your
child a drink or a lollipop to suck on during takeoff and
landing (with infants you can breast-feed or use a bottle)
to minimize the effect of pressure changes in the middle
ear and to help reduce the risk of spontaneous fluid accumulation in the middle ear. Decongestant nose drops taken
twenty minutes before takeoff and landing may also help the
eustachian tube to function better during the plane's ascent
and descent.

## Ventilating the Middle Ear

Before the advent of tympanostomy tubes (tubes inserted
in the eardrum to ventilate the middle ear, see Chapter 5) doctors treating children with otitis media with effusion (OME)

sometimes would teach them special techniques to ventilate the middle ear. The techniques are simple, such as swallowing while pinching the nostrils shut, which forces air into the middle ear and produces a popping sensation. Performing these maneuvers three times a day for several weeks may help promote drainage of fluid from the middle ear. A few doctors still recommend practicing these techniques to help prevent initial buildup of fluid. If you are interested in trying such methods with your child, check with your doctor first to see whether he thinks it would be appropriate for your child and for more details on performing the different techniques. There are also some precautions if your child practices the maneuvers.

- Ear ventilation maneuvers should *not* be used while your child has a cold; such a practice could force bacteria or viruses into the middle ear.

- The techniques are appropriate only for children who are four years or older.

- In order for these techniques to have any effect, they need to be done three times a day over several weeks during periods when you think your child is susceptible to ear infections.

## Addressing Risk Factors

You may have little control over many of the risk factors associated with ear infections such as heredity, race, and gender (see Chapter 2), but there are three key factors, which, if controlled adequately during the periods when your child is most vulnerable to infection, can greatly reduce your child's chances of acquiring ear infections.

## Tobacco Smoke

Eliminating exposure to tobacco smoke is a crucial step in protecting all children from ear infections. Secondhand cigarette smoke is estimated to be one of the main causes of eustachian tube dysfunction in some children (see Chapter 2). Some ways to limit exposure to secondhand smoke are as follows:

- If possible, do not permit smoking in your home. If any members of your household smoke, ask them to smoke outside. Confining smoking to one room that your child does not use is not an adequate preventive measure, as secondhand smoke will still spread to other rooms in the house.
- If secondhand smoke is unavoidable, consider using a portable air-cleaning device; be aware, however, that the effectiveness of these devices depends on the size of the room and the volume of smoke needed to be removed. Many units are now rated by the clean air delivery rate (CADR), which is helpful in selecting the correct size unit for a particular room.
- Filling a room with three or four houseplants may help reduce the effects of secondhand smoke; plants are not advised, however, for children with allergies to mold (see page 208).
- Heavy smokers should clean their clothing frequently to eliminate smoke residue.
- When outside the home, keep your child away from any enclosed smoking areas and do not permit smoking in your car, even with the windows open. If you cannot avoid a public venue where people are smoking, try to stay near an open window or door to minimize the effects of secondhand smoke.

Obviously, the best answer is to be firm about family members stopping smoking and to not allow any smoking in your home. This is the healthiest choice for all members of your household.

## Breast-Feeding Versus Formula Feeding

Breast-feeding is one of the best ways to build your child's immune system and protect against ear infections. Breast milk supplies babies with their mother's antibodies (substances that fight infection). A specific type of antibody, called immunoglobulin IgA, attaches to the lining of the ears, nose, and throat to protect your child against many of the bacteria that cause ear infections. Breast milk also contains a protein called lactoferrin and enzymes called lysosomes that are effective at killing several types of bacteria. Several studies have found that children who were formula-fed were more likely to get ear infections than children who were breast-fed, but these findings may be due to the angle at which feeding occurs when bottle-feeding rather than because of the actual composition of the formula.

If a mother is able to breast-feed her child (and feels comfortable doing so), she should do so for at least the first three months; the protective benefits may extend for much longer. If a mother has to be away from her child during the day because of professional commitments, she may want to pump her milk so that a caregiver can give her child breast milk during the day. Or if a child is old enough, she can be fed solid foods during the day, and continue to nurse in the evening when her mother is home.

In addition, try to limit the amount of formula you give to your child during the first three to six months of life; the American Academy of Pediatrics recommends that children should receive breast milk for the first year. Formula is made from soy or cow's milk protein and these foreign proteins lack the protective mechanisms of breast milk.

## Day Care

To reduce the risk of exposure to viral and bacterial infections that can lead to ear infections, try to avoid putting your child in day care, at least during the winter seasons when she is under two years of age. If you have no other option regarding child care, there are a few ways you can minimize the risks for ear infections associated with day care.

- Choose a care situation with six or fewer children.

- Avoid a home or facility with pets, rugs, or smoking, especially if your child has allergies.

- During the winter season, when your child is between six and twenty-four months of age, try to arrange for an at-home caregiver, even a few days a week, if possible.

- Ask the day care provider to notify you if another child at the facility seems to be sick; you can always make the decision to bring your child home that day.

# Treating Colds

Colds are the most common ailment in children under age five and ear infections frequently follow a cold. While it is difficult to stop the numerous viruses that can cause colds (see Chapter 2), there are several things you can do to minimize the effects of a cold on your child, thus reducing the risk that the cold will lead to an ear infection. Remember that antibiotics do not work against viral infections, and antihistamines and decongestants have not been shown to be very effective in relieving cold symptoms in children under five years of age (see Chapter 4). However, there are many practical, simple, commonsense steps you can take to treat your child's cold.

## Rest

Make sure your child gets plenty of rest. Sleep is an important part of the healing process. Though sleeping through the night may be difficult for your child because she is congested, frequent naps during the day can help make up the difference in lost sleep. You can allow your child to undertake only mild activity, such as playing cards or other games if she starts getting restless, but restrict any vigorous physical activity. The added stress on the body during work or play makes it more difficult for the body to fight infection.

## Fluids

During a cold, viruses cause excess fluids to be secreted in the lining of the nose, so it is important to make sure your child is getting adequate fluids. Drinking water, nonherbal, decaffeinated teas, Pedialyte, Gatorade, and broth are good ways to replenish your child's fluids. The frequent swallowing may also "exercise" the eustachian tubes.

## Saltwater (Saline) Nose Drops

Saline drops are used to thin out the mucus, clear excess

fluid, and decrease congestion and coughing. Using saline nose drops four to five times a day is one of the best ways to relieve your child's cold symptoms. Gently squirt the drops into both nostrils, holding your child's head slightly back, then set your child upright and use a bulb aspirator to suck the fluid back out. Saline drops can be bought at most pharmacies. You can also make drops at home using 1/4 teaspoon of salt in 8 ounces of warm water. Using kosher salt is preferable if possible, since it has fewer or no additional minerals and is more pure. If making the solution at home, you should mix a fresh batch daily.

## Elevating the Head

Elevating your child's head, by propping it up on pillows when she is lying down, helps to keep the airway passages clear and allows a natural drainage of fluid to occur, especially in children who have upper respiratory infections. Encourage her to sit up in bed as much as possible when she is awake. For infants lying in their crib, you can prop up one end of the crib to keep their head slightly elevated.

## Nose Blowing

Frequent nose blowing helps to keep the air passages clear and to reduce dripping of mucus down the throat (postnasal drip), which can irritate the throat and cause coughing. You can help your child to gently blow, keeping one of her nostrils open at all times. Avoid any forceful blowing of the nose while both nostrils or the mouth is closed since this may cause bacteria or viruses to be blown into the middle ear. If your child is too young to blow her nose, you can use a rubber bulb aspirator to gently suck the mucus out. Squeeze the bulb gently, insert it in one nostril, then release it quickly to draw the fluid out.

## Inhaling Steam

Inhaling steam is helpful for easing congestion, particularly if your child has mucus in her chest, characterized by a "wet" or phlegm-filled cough, or has croup (noisy, difficult breathing distinguished by a barking cough). To have your child inhale steam you can use the following methods:

- Use a vaporizer at night to increase the amount of moisture in her bedroom.
- If your child is five years of age or older, you can fill a bowl with hot water, make a tent over it with a towel, and let your child inhale the steam for ten to fifteen minutes.
- For a younger child, you can create steam in the bathroom by turning on the hot water taps and leaving the door closed for a while. Then sit in the bathroom with your child, letting her inhale the steam. (You should *not* leave your child alone in the bathroom.) Once your child has inhaled the steam, lay her on her stomach and gently pat her back to help break up the mucus in the lungs.

## Other Measures

There are a few other steps you can undertake in caring for your child's cold. These measures may help relieve your child's symptoms during a cold, but there is not conclusive evidence that they are effective for treating colds in children. However, they can do no harm to your child and may offer some extra help.

### Vitamin C

Research suggests that vitamin C is helpful for treating colds in adults (but not necessarily in preventing colds). If you want to give your child vitamin C when she has a cold, the best source is fresh orange juice and other citrus fruits. If you wish to give your child vitamin supplements instead, make sure the supplements are appropriate for children (some are made specifically for infants and toddlers). In addition, try to find a supplement that contains mineral-ascorbate-buffered vitamin C and no sugar.

### Zinc

Zinc has been found to help to relieve symptoms of a cold in adults. If you want to try zinc for your child's cold, use preparations made specifically for children; lozenges are usually the best form if your child is old enough to suck on them. In addition, do not exceed the recommended dosage for your child; excess zinc can cause abdominal discomfort and nausea.

### Herbal Remedies

If you want to try an herbal remedy when your child has a cold, echinacea is considered safe for children and it has little risk of side effects (see Chapter 6). Research indicates that echinacea can help the recovery process if given at the first sign of a cold. When buying echinacea, select drops (tinctures) that are made specifically for children and follow the dosage instructions for your child's age. Echinacea does not have a pleasant taste, so it is a good idea to give it to your child by putting the drops in juice or warm tea or broth. Echinacea should only be given on a daily basis for one to two weeks when your child has a cold. Follow the manufacturer's recommendations for dose and duration.

*Homeopathic Medicines*

Homeopathic medicines are safe for young children and have little risk of side effects (see Chapter 6). There are several homeopathic medicines designed to relieve specific symptoms of cold, including:

- Kali muriacticum—to relieve nasal congestion and swollen glands

- Potassium chloride—for runny nose and cough

- Mercurous chloride—for phlegm and swollen adenoids

There are also "combination" remedies, containing three to eight medicines, that are designed to relieve several symptoms of cold (although many homeopathic doctors recommend a single medicine for more effective relief). Consult with a knowledgeable pharmacist or reputable manual to select the medicine that is most appropriate, based on your child's specific symptoms; you may also want to check with your doctor, especially if he is familiar with homeopathic remedies. Within the dosage guidelines for your child's age, you can give her the medicine more frequently initially when her symptoms are more severe. In addition, if your child's symptoms worsen or do not improve in five to seven days, you should consult with your doctor.

# Treating Allergies

If your child is showing signs of allergies—continually runny nose, red, watery, itchy eyes, or wheezing (tightness in the chest when breathing)—check with your doctor about consulting a specialist trained to treat allergies (an allergist).

Treating your child's allergies may greatly reduce her chances of getting ear infections as some studies have shown that children with persistent or recurrent ear infections often have some type of allergic condition (see Chapter 2).

The allergist will evaluate your child's antibody function and also identify substances causing allergic reactions through blood tests and skin-prick tests (however, formal allergy testing of children younger than three years of age is currently felt to be unreliable). If your child is found to have specific allergies, you can take steps to remove household irritants (see below) and limit your child's exposure to outdoor allergens. If your child is found to be allergic to certain foods, eliminating these foods from her daily diet is also recommended (see below).

As noted above, allergies may be difficult to reliably diagnose in very young children (under three years of age). But even if your child's allergy tests are inconclusive, you may find that eliminating common irritants in the home or reducing intake of certain foods, particularly dairy products, can have a beneficial effect on your child.

## Eliminating Household Irritants

If your child has tested positive to specific allergens, it is important to do as much as possible to eliminate these substances in your home. Following are a few basic guidelines for ridding your home of irritants. You can also consult with your allergist for further preventive strategies.

### Dust

It is a real challenge trying to keep a home dust free; it requires almost daily effort to maintain such an environment. But for a child who is allergic to dust, it is well worth the effort. You should dust surfaces of your child's room with a damp cloth daily and vacuum a few times a week if possible. In selecting a vacuum cleaner, choose a model that is designed to remove allergens. (Some vacuums suck up dirt but put the allergens back into the air.)

To make your job easier and to reduce irritants for your child, you can also take the following steps:

- Remove any carpets or rugs from your child's room; use wood or vinyl flooring instead.

- Keep stuffed animals out of the child's bedroom and give your child wooden or plastic toys; any cloth toys that are kept should be washed frequently. Stuffed animals can stay in a playroom.

- Avoid items that collect dust easily, such as venetian blinds.

- Use plastic casing (underneath the sheets and pillowcases) for your child's mattress and pillows; use only washable cotton blankets and sheets on the bed.

- During winter months, change the furnace filter periodically to reduce dust particles in the air; a humidifier may also help to reduce dust in the air.

- Use a portable air-cleaning device in your child's room.

### Mold

While dust is a visible allergen in the home, mold is often unseen, but is just as much an irritant for children with mold allergies. To rid your home of mold you can take the following steps:

- Clean areas that retain moisture (such as the bathroom) frequently with disinfectant.

- If any rooms in your home have damp walls, apply a coat of mold-inhibiting paint, available at most hardware stores.

- Control dampness in a room by using a dehumidifier.

- Spray your dehumidifier, air conditioner, or air vents, regularly with disinfectant to prevent mold from growing in them.

- Make sure clothing and shoes dry completely after being washed; damp items are a source of mold.

- Remove houseplants from any areas where your child plays since they may contain mold.

### Pet Dander

Dander is loose scales that form on the skin and shed from the coat of various animals such as dogs and cats. (It does not matter whether the animal's hair is long or short.) If your child has tested allergic to pet dander, you may want to reconsider a decision to keep pets, if you already have them. For some children, removal of pets from the home is the only way to improve their allergic condition. If you decide to try more moderate measures first, keep the pet out of the area where your child sleeps, confine the pet to one room of the house, keep the pet outside whenever possible, and vacuum regularly in areas where your pet has been. You should brush the animal's coat and bathe your pet regularly to eliminate excess dander, but all grooming should be done outside of the house and away from any area where your child plays.

## A Personal Experience:
## A Persistent Cold

After three months of what seemed like a never-ending cold, David took his five-year-old son, Jonathan, to the pediatrician. David explained to the doctor that Jonathan's cold was usually mild and was not accompanied by a fever, but that he was concerned about the persistence of the symptoms. His son had not missed any school and was in good spirits, although sometimes he had difficulty sleeping because his nose was stuffy at night.

The doctor examined Jonathan and asked him and his father about the illness and whether anything new had happened at home. Were there any new pets or changes in day care? David related that about three months ago they had moved into a fifty-year-old house. The house was in fairly good shape, although there had been some water damage and mold in the basement, which they had cleaned up. David also remembered that his son's cold had gone away when he had taken a five-day trip to his grandmother's house, only to return when he came home. The doctor explained that it was possible that Jonathan was having an allergic reaction to mold spores that remained in the house and recommended that his son be examined by an allergist. He also gave David some literature, which described ways to reduce mold and improve air quality in the home.

*Down*

If your child is allergic to down, she should not use any pillows, comforters, or clothing that contain any type of down (such as duck down or goose down). Your child's pillows should be of synthetic fibers and comforters should be of washable cotton.

## Elimination Diet

If your child has tested positive for allergies to specific foods, then it is important to eliminate those foods from her diet. In studies of children with recurrent otitis media with effusion (OME) who were also found to be allergic to certain foods, there was a significant improvement in their condition when they stayed away from the food items over a four- to five-month period of time.

It can be challenging to eliminate items from your child's diet, particularly common foods such as milk. Fortunately, there are many alternative products available for children who have specific food allergies: soy and rice milk can replace cow's milk; almond or cashew butters can replace peanut butter; for children allergic to wheat there are cereals, bread, and baked goods available in wheat-free varieties. In addition, check the ingredient label on any foods you buy to make sure that they do not contain substances to which your child is allergic.

## Checking for Cow's Milk Allergies

If your child has not yet been tested for allergies, but you suspect that she may be allergic to cow's milk, there is a preliminary way to check your child's reaction to dairy prod-

ucts. Eliminate milk and all dairy products from her diet for
one week, then on the eighth day give your child several
glasses of milk. If you notice a reaction in your child
(increased congestion, sneezing), there is a chance that she
is allergic to milk, and you might want to consult with your
doctor about allergy testing.

## Checking for Food Allergies Early On

For infants just starting on solid foods at four to six
months of age, doctors recommend starting with one food
(such as rice cereal), then introducing one new food every
three to four days and checking whether it causes any reaction. This method provides a useful way to discover any
potential food allergies early on. Some foods are associated
with allergic reactions more than others, and doctors recommend that these foods—particularly eggs, citrus fruit, fish,
and peanuts and peanut products—should be avoided until
the child is over one year of age. In fact, peanuts should be
avoided until the age of four years, when the child's teeth
and oral motor coordination have matured enough to
decrease the likelihood of choking.

## Medications

Medications—both conventional and alternative—are
also available for children who are allergic to airborne substances such as pollen.

### Conventional Medications

Antihistamines—both prescription and over-the-counter
medications—are commonly used to treat symptoms of

allergies. These medications often have adverse effects (see Chapter 4). However, newer antihistamines minimize such effects. For example, the antihistamines loratadine (sold under the brand name Claritin) and fexofenadine (Allegra) are prescription drugs designed to relieve seasonal allergies without causing significant drowsiness, but are only safe for children over six years of age. Cetirizine (Zyrtec), a prescription antihistamine approved for children two years of age and older, had few side effects in clinical studies with children. Consult with your doctor (and also the allergist, if you are seeing one) as to which medications would be appropriate for your child.

### Alternative Therapies

Homeopathic medicines and herbal remedies (see Chapter 6) have also been used to treat allergies. If you are interested in pursuing alternative treatments for your child's allergies, it is advisable to make an appointment with a naturopathic doctor who specializes in homeopathy (see Chapter 7). While you may be able to select herbal or homeopathic products on your own that help to relieve your child's symptoms, treating chronic conditions such as allergies with alternative therapies requires the guidance of a qualified and experienced alternative practitioner. Additionally, some herbal products are not recommended for use in children or infants—so it is important to be careful when selecting herbal remedies for your child.

## Immunotherapy

Immunotherapy (allergy shots) is another option for children (over the age of three years) who are allergic to airborne substances. Immunotherapy involves a series of injections (usually weekly or biweekly) that stimulate the production of a "blocking" antibody (immunoglobulin type IgG) that protects the child when she is exposed to the specific allergen(s). If controlling household irritants is not having much of an effect on your child's allergic condition, and your child is not responding to medications, you may want to consult with the allergist to see whether allergy shots are an appropriate option for your child.

Nine

# Parenting the Child
# with Ear Infections

Parenting is always a uniquely rewarding but challenging endeavor, and parenting a child with ear infections requires an extra bit of stamina and determination at times. But you should feel reassured that by comforting your child during the infection, seeking medical attention when needed, and monitoring your child after treatment, you are doing the best job possible to care for your child.

Helping to relieve your child's symptoms when she has an ear infection is an important part of your parental role. In addition, providing psychological and emotional support to your child can boost her spirits and help recovery. Reassure your child that you will take care of her and that she will get better soon. Spend extra time with your child when she is sick and stay up with her during her sleepless nights to help her feel safe and secure. Other measures—such as preparing your child to see the doctor or making special arrangements with her babysitter, day care, or school—can also help your child to get through her infection and resume her normal schedule of activities upon recovery.

# Preparing Your Child to See the Doctor

Toddlers and slightly older children may feel a little anxious before visiting the doctor—whether they are healthy or sick—especially if they previously had an unpleasant experience at the doctor (such as receiving a vaccination). Anxiety is a normal part of children's mental and emotional preparation for an unknown or potentially scary event. As a parent, there are many ways you can help prepare your child for seeing the doctor, both during well-care visits and appointments due to ear infections. The following suggestions offer a few ideas for how to help make a trip to the doctor seem

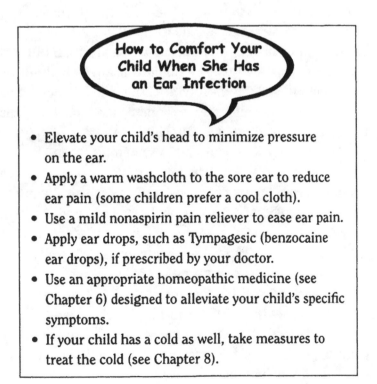

### How to Comfort Your Child When She Has an Ear Infection

- Elevate your child's head to minimize pressure on the ear.
- Apply a warm washcloth to the sore ear to reduce ear pain (some children prefer a cool cloth).
- Use a mild nonaspirin pain reliever to ease ear pain.
- Apply ear drops, such as Tympagesic (benzocaine ear drops), if prescribed by your doctor.
- Use an appropriate homeopathic medicine (see Chapter 6) designed to alleviate your child's specific symptoms.
- If your child has a cold as well, take measures to treat the cold (see Chapter 8).

more like an adventure for your child and less like a reason for worry. Of course, every child is different, so you should assess what approaches might be most appropriate for your child—based on her age and her personality—and also come up with further strategies of your own. In addition, if your child has to undergo surgery (see Chapter 5), you can build on some of these methods and use additional ones to help your child prepare for the procedure.

## Well-Care Visits

Preparing your child for routine well-child checkups with the doctor might make it a little easier when you have to bring her in because of a possible ear infection.

### Read Books

To help your child understand what a visit to the doctor is all about, you can read her stories about going to the doctor (a list of books is provided in the Resources section). One mother read different books to her child each night for a week, with the result that her child was excited to visit the doctor so that she could see for herself all of the things that she had heard about in the books.

### Play Games

To prepare your child for a checkup, you can play games with her. Most children love to play doctor, trying out a toy stethoscope. One parent pretended to conduct an examination on her child, then she let her child do a pretend examnation on her. When they went to the doctor's office, the doctor conducted a quick "practice" exam on the parent while the child watched; then the child was ready for her turn.

*Combine a Visit to the Doctor with a Special Outing*

You can do something special with your child before or after she has had her doctor's appointment, such as taking her to a playground or out for a meal. Your child may begin to associate doctor's visits with fun events rather than with illness.

## Visits for Ear Infections

Visiting the doctor for an ear infection involves a special set of considerations. Your child will not be feeling well, she may be experiencing pain, and you may not have much time to prepare her for a visit. Hopefully your child has had a few well-care visits that were pleasant experiences, so she will not feel excessively anxious about seeing the doctor. In addition, you can do a few extra things to help prepare her for the visit.

### Reassure Your Child

Reassure your child that you will be with her for the whole time at the appointment. Explain to your child that the doctor will find out why she is not feeling well and what will make her feel better.

### Engage Her Imagination

Engage your child's imagination in explaining that something is wrong with her ear. Fantastical images might appeal to some children, such as the notion one doctor uses during pneumatic otoscopy of looking for Big Bird in the child's ear and "blowing him a kiss." Dr. Seuss's *One Fish Two Fish Red Fish Blue Fish* has a wonderfully playful rhyme about a bird in the ear. Such images can help a young child understand that there is something "funny" with her ear, and the doctor will try to fix it.

### Explain What Will Happen During the Exam

For slightly older children, you can describe to them in simple terms some of the tests the doctor might conduct during the visit. You can also give your child an idea of what the eardrum is like by using a toy drum with the drumskin stretched tight across the top.

If you think it will not scare your child, you can explain that a few things (such as the doctor clearing away excess wax in the ear canal) might hurt a tiny bit, but just for a moment. (With most children it is helpful to give them a little warning so they will not be taken by surprise during the exam.) But give your child an idea of what the momentary pain might compare to, such as pulling an adhesive bandage off quickly, so that she will not be too worried about the pain.

### Minimize Your Own Feelings of Worry

If you find *yourself* feeling a little anxious about the visit (perhaps you are worried about your child being diagnosed with another ear infection), try not to let your stress show. Your child will sense your mood and it may affect her reactions as well. It is never useful to say something like, "I hope the doctor stops hurting you soon."

### Stay Calm and Patient During the Exam

Do not feel frustrated if the doctor's visit does not go smoothly even after your preparations. Sometimes children will start fussing and crying during an ear examination and the best thing parents and doctors can do is to be gentle, patient, and comforting. It is important not to feel bad if your child cries during the exam; doctors are accustomed to crying and do not attribute it to poor parenting. Your doctor can also take extra steps to help make the visit easier for your child.

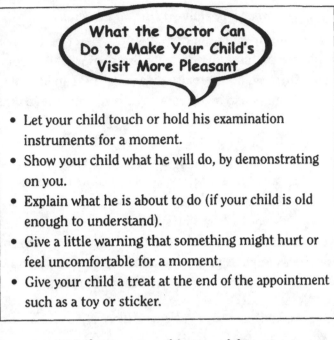

- Let your child touch or hold his examination instruments for a moment.
- Show your child what he will do, by demonstrating on you.
- Explain what he is about to do (if your child is old enough to understand).
- Give a little warning that something might hurt or feel uncomfortable for a moment.
- Give your child a treat at the end of the appointment such as a toy or sticker.

# When to Keep Your Child Out of School

If your child is showing signs of a potential ear infection—fever, ear pain, irritability, sleeplessness—it is a good idea to keep her home from school (or day care) to see whether the symptoms subside. If the symptoms do not subside, you will need to see the doctor for diagnosis and treatment. Once the doctor has seen your child and prescribed a treatment, ask him when it would be appropriate to allow your child to resume her school activities. Ear infections are not contagious, so your child cannot infect other children in her class. However, if your child's symptoms change for the worse or become more severe, contact your doctor and inform him of the changes; such changes could signal that the treatment is not working.

When you are bringing your child back to school after she has had an ear infection, it is important to restrict her exposure to other children that may have colds, flu, or other viral infections (the viruses that cause such infections are easily contracted in close quarters such as a classroom). Check with your child's teacher to make sure that there are no children in the class with visible signs of cold or flu before letting your child return to class.

# Instructions for Your Caregiver When Your Child Is Home Sick

If at all possible you (your spouse or partner or a close family member or friend that your child is accustomed to spending time with) should stay home with your child during the first few days of the ear infection when the symptoms are more severe—either while waiting a few days to see the doctor, or after she has received treatment from the doctor. Knowing that a parent or close relative or friend is nearby will reduce your child's stress in coping with the illness.

Once your child's symptoms have diminished somewhat, you can arrange for additional caregivers or baby-sitters if needed. (Day care is not appropriate until your child is feeling better.) If your child normally has a sitter, she should feel comfortable under your sitter's care, with adequate reassurance from you that you will not be away from her for long. But if your child is normally at school or with friends while you are at work, an at-home caregiver may be a big adjustment for her.

You should leave clear, written instructions with your baby-sitter (or anyone else who is watching your child) regarding special care for your child while you are away, including information about medications, rest, fluids, and monitoring of your child and including your and your doctor's phone number (see also Monitoring, below).

## Medications

Make sure that your sitter understands the proper dosage for the medication, the appropriate time to give it, whether to give it with food or liquids, and how to store it (some liquid antibiotics require refrigeration). Let your sitter know about any possible side effects of the medication, and instruct her regarding how to notify you if she sees any adverse reaction (see below).

## Rest

You should let the caregiver know that it is important for your child to rest; she should not let your child undertake any vigorous physical activity. Leave plenty of books, cards, and games to help the sitter keep your child occupied with low-energy-level activities.

## Fluids

Leave plenty of water, nonherbal decaffeinated teas, and broth in the house and ask your sitter to encourage your child to drink as frequently as possible. Some juices can cause diarrhea, so they may not be recommended when a child is sick or taking an antibiotic.

## Monitoring

Your child's caregiver should be told about signs that warrant a call to you, such as a fever that suddenly rises or ear pain that becomes severe. You should always leave a phone number with your sitter where you can be reached. You may also want to ask a relative or friend to be backup support, on the off chance that your sitter cannot reach you by phone.

In addition, you should leave the name and phone number of your child's doctor, a number to call for emergency services, as well as your child's health insurance information in the rare instance that it might be necessary for your sitter to seek immediate medical attention for your child. (The sitter should contact emergency services first, then call you.) While your sitter will most likely never need to use this information, it is a wise precaution to undertake. Some parents leave a medical release form as well, granting permission for medical assistance to be given in their absence.

# What to Do When Your Child Is Away

Whether your child is returning to school or to a day care situation after having an ear infection, there are a few arrangements you can undertake that will make her transition back to her normal routine easier.

## Medications

If your child is going back to school (or day care), it is important to check with the school administration or day care facility about arrangements regarding your child's medications; if your child is on a medication that is only needed twice a day, such special arrangements may not be necessary.

Schools have different policies in regard to giving medications. If your school allows administration of your child's medicines, find out when the nurse (or other personnel) is able to dispense medicines for your child. You should also provide written instructions on dosage, storage, and side effects of your child's medicine. If your child is older and has antibiotic chewable tablets or other types of medications that she can take herself, it may suffice to arrange a simple reminder from her teacher or school nurse of the appropriate time to take the medicine.

Many schools, however, *do not* allow medication to be given to children at school; some schools might not even allow a child to carry in her own medicines. If it is not possible for your child to be given her medicine at school, check with your doctor about modifying the dosage schedule so that she can receive medications immediately before and after school.

In addition, you should leave information with the teacher or day care facility about your child's doctor and where you can be reached that day. Many schools have such information on file already, but it is a good idea to provide it directly to your child's teacher as a backup measure.

## Physical Activities

After your child has been at home resting for three to four days while recovering from her ear infection, it is a good idea to limit her physical activities at school at least for another two to three days, or until she is feeling fully strong again. You can ask your doctor his opinion and also get a note from the doctor if it is necessary to excuse your child from recreation or gym exercises, but generally once your child is feeling well, you will not have to restrict her activity. Some doctors also recommend restricting swimming for at least the ten days that antibiotic treatment is being given. In general, however, water exposure or swimming only needs to be avoided when there is a perforation of the eardrum. If this condition does not exist, swimming does not need to be restricted.

## Adjusting for Temporary Hearing Impairment

Even if your child is feeling better, she may still have some fluid in her ears for a few weeks or more, which may cause some mild temporary hearing loss (see Chapter 1). It is a good idea to let your child's teacher know about this possible impairment so he can make adjustments if necessary for your child to sit closer to the front of the classroom. If one ear is affected more than the other, your child can sit at a slight angle with her better ear close to the teacher. The teacher can also help by facing your child when he speaks to her and making sure that distracting background noises are kept to a minimum. In addition, ask the teacher to tell you if he notices any differences in your child's behavior or in her progress at school and to alert you to any possible changes in your child's hearing ability.

# Final Words of Encouragement

We hope that after reading this book and other publications, talking to friends, and consulting with your doctor, you feel more confident and positive about managing your child's ear infections. You can feel empowered by being able to recognize signs of ear infection, prepare for your child's visit to the doctor, discuss treatment options, and monitor your child's progress to full recovery.

If you have to confront an ear infection in your child in the near future, here are a few final reminders to help you through the experience.

- Remember that most ear infections resolve on their own and there are very few cases of serious problems resulting from ear infections. Permanent hearing loss is very uncommon following ear infections.
- There are usually several options for treating ear infections—including simple monitoring and observation—and you can work together with your doctor to decide on the treatment plan that is best for your child.
- You are a very important part of your child's health care team. In discussing your child's care with your doctor, trust your instincts, ask questions, seek additional information, and be open and honest about your opinions.
- Remember, you and your doctor share the same goal—a happy, healthy child.

Finally remember that your child *will* outgrow her vulnerability to ear infections, and that the sleepless nights due to ear pain will eventually seem like a distant memory.

# Resources

## Books for Parents

Fugh-Berman, A. *Alternative Medicine—What Works.* Baltimore: Williams & Wilkins, 1997.

Greene, A. R. *The Parent's Complete Guide to Ear Infections.* Allentown, Penn.: People's Medical Society, 1997.

Grundfast, K., and Carney, C. *Ear Infections in Your Child.* New York: Warner Books, 1987.

Mindell, E. *Earl Mindell's New Herb Bible.* New York: Simon & Schuster, 1999.

Offit, P., Fass-Offit, B., and Bell, L. *Breaking the Antibiotic Habit. A Parent's Guide to Coughs, Colds, Ear Infections, and Sore Throats.* New York: John Wiley & Sons, 1999.

Schmidt, M. A. *Healing Childhood Ear Infections.* Berkeley, Calif.: North Atlantic Books, 1999.

Zand, J. *Smart Medicine for a Healthier Child.* Wayne, N.J.: Avery Publishing Group, 1994.

## Books for Children

Berenstain, Stan, and Berenstain, Jan. *The Berenstain Bears Go to the Doctor.* New York: Random House, 1981.

Elliott, Ingrid Glatz. *Hospital Roadmap.* Resources for Children in Hospitals, 1982.

Hautzig, Debra, and Elliott, Dan. *A Visit to the Sesame Street Hospital: Featuring Jim Henson's Sesame Street Muppets.* New York: Random House, 1985.

Lansky, Vicki. *Koko Bear's Big Earache: Preparing Your Child for Ear Tube Surgery.* Minnetonka, Minn.: Book Peddlers, 1990.

Oxenbury, Helen. *The Checkup.* New York: Dial Books, 1983.

Rey, Margaret. *Curious George Goes to the Hospital.* Boston: Houghton Mifflin, 1966.

Rogers, Fred. *Going to the Hospital.* New York: Putnam, 1997.

Dr. Seuss. *One Fish Two Fish Red Fish Blue Fish.* New York: Random House, 1976.

## Organizations, Associations, and Web Sites

### General Information on Health and Ear Infections

Agency for Healthcare Research and Quality
Department of Health and Human Services
Web site: www.ahrq.gov/clinic/cpgonline.htm for
Clinical Practice Guideline No. 12, Otitis Media with
Effusion (professional guideline) and Middle Ear Fluid
in Young Children (consumer version)

American Academy of Family Physicians (AAFP)
11400 Tomahawk Creek Pathway
Leawood, KS 66211
Phone: 913-906-6000
Web site: www.aafp.org

American Academy of Otolaryngology—Head and Neck
Surgery (AAO-HNS)
One Prince Street
Alexandria, VA 22314
Phone: 703-836-4444
Web site: www.entnet.org

American Academy of Pediatrics (AAP)
National Headquarters
141 Northwest Point Boulevard
Elk Grove Village, IL 60007
Phone: 847-434-4000, Fax: 847-434-8000
Web site: www.aap.org

American Board of Pediatrics (ABP)
111 Silver Cedar Court
Chapel Hill, NC 27514
Phone: 919-929-0461, Fax: 919-929-9255
Web site: www.abp.org

American Medical Association (AMA)
515 North State Street
Chicago, IL 60610
Phone: 312-464-5000
Web site: www.ama-assn.org

Centers for Disease Control and Prevention (CDC)
1600 Clifton Rd.
Atlanta, GA 30333
Phone: 800-311-3435
Web site: www.cdc.gov

National Institutes of Health (NIH)
Bethesda, MD 20892
Web site: www.nih.gov
See also National Center of Complementary and Alternative
Medicine, National Institute of Allergy and Infectious Diseases, and
National Institute on Deafness and Other Communication Disorders.

## Allergies

American Academy of Allergy, Asthma and Immunology (AAAAI)
611 East Wells Street
Milwaukee, WI 53202
Phone: 800-822-2762
Web site: www.aaaai.org

National Institute of Allergy and Infectious Diseases (NIAID)
National Institutes of Health
NIAID Office of Communications and Public Liaison
Building 31, Room 7A-50
31 Center Drive MSC 2520
Bethesda, MD 20892
Web site: www.niaid.nih.gov

## Alternative Therapies

American Association of Naturopathic Physicians (AANP)
8201 Greensboro Drive, Suite 300
McClean, VA 22102
Phone: 703-610-9037, Fax: 703-610-9005
Web site: www.aanp.net

American Chiropractic Association (ACA)
1701 Clarendon Blvd.
Arlington, VA 22209
Phone: 800-986-4636, Fax: 703-243-2593
Web site: www.amerchiro.org

Chiroweb.com
www.chiroweb.com
Web site with many chiropractic links; the following
publication is available free on this site at
www.chiroweb.com/archives/ahcpr/uschiros.htm

Chiropractic in the United States: Training, Practice, and
Research. Agency for Health Care Policy and Research,
AHCPR Publication No. 98-N002,
December 1997

Herb Research Foundation (HRF)
1007 Pearl St. Suite 200
Boulder, CO 80302
Phone: 303-449-2265, Fax: 303-449-7849
Voice mail: 800-748-2617
Web site: www.herbs.org

Homeopathic Academy of Naturopathic Physicians
(HANP)
12132 SE Forster Place
Portland, OR 97266
Phone: 503-761-3298, Fax: 503-762-1929
Web site: www.healthy.net/pan/pa/homeopathic/hanp

International Chiropractors Association (ICA)
1110 N. Glebe Rd., Suite 1000
Arlington, VA 22201
Phone: 800-423-4690, Fax: 703-528-5023
Web site: www.chiropractic.org

National Center for Alternative and Complementary Medicine
(NCCAM)
NCCAM Clearinghouse
PO Box 8218

Silver Spring, MD 20907
Phone: 888-644-6226, Fax: 301-495-4957
Web site: http://nccam.nih.gov

## Antibiotic Use

US Food and Drug Administration (FDA)
Phone: 1-888-463-6332
Web site: www.fda.gov

## Hearing Impairment

American Speech-Language-Hearing Association (ASHA)
10801 Rockville Pike
Rockville, MD 20852
Phone: 301-897-5700, Fax: 301-897-7355
Web site: www.asha.org

Boystown National Research Hospital
555 North 30th St.
Omaha, NE 68131
Phone: 402-498-6749
Web site: www.boystown.org/btnrh/

National Institute on Deafness and Other Communication
Disorders (NIDCD)
National Institutes of Health
31 Center Drive MSC 2320
Bethesda, MD 20892
Phone: 301-496-7243, Fax: 301-402-0018
Web site: www.nih.gov/nidcd/

## Physician Certification

American Board of Medical Specialties
(ABMS)
1007 Church Street, Suite 404
Evanston, IL 60201
Phone: 847-491-9091, Fax: 847-328-3596
Web site: www.abms.org

# Index

acetaminophen, 58, 97, 100, 101
aconite, 148
acoustic reflectometry, 63
acute (suppurative) otitis media (AOM),
    18–20, 22–23, 30, 162–63
    causes of, 33–36, 38, 43, 89, 163
    diagnosis of, 60, 66
    follow-up for, 25, 78–79
    recurrence of, 21, 27, 42–49, 90,
        98, 107, 112–13, 114, 123,
        162–63
    symptoms of, 19–20, 162
    treatment of, 20, 35, 81, 97–98,
        107, 113, 114, 123–24, 159, 163
    viral infections and, 192
acute serous otitis media, see otitis media
    with effusion
adenoidectomy, 23, 37, 47, 123–30
    benefits and limitations of, 130
    follow-up for, 127–29
    indicators for, 123–24
    possible complications of, 129–30
    procedure for, 125–27
    tonsillectomy combined with, 131
adenoids, 13, 16, 23, 35, 37, 48
    chronic infection of, 46–47, 164
advocacy for your child, 178–80
age of child:
    antibiotics and, 91
    of onset of infection, 52
    as risk factor, 50–51
Agency for Health Care Policy and
    Research (AHCPR), 98, 100, 102,
    104
airplane travel, 197
air pressure, 12, 197
allergies, 7, 18, 21, 22, 23, 32, 33, 35,
    38–39, 43, 67, 68, 102, 107, 120,
    164, 199, 201, 229
    to antibiotics, 92–93, 94
    to foods, 39, 207, 211–12
    to formula, 55
    to herbal remedies, 139
    treatment of, 206–14
allergy shots, 39, 213–14
allergy testing, 39, 207
alternative treatments, see complemen-
    tary and alternative medicine
American ginseng, 142, 144

Amoxil, see amoxicillin
amoxicillin, 43, 44, 86, 89–90, 91, 96
amoxicillin-clavulanate, 86, 90, 91, 96
analgesics, 100–101
anatomy of ear, 9–13
anesthesia, general, 113, 114, 116–18,
    121, 125–27, 130
antibiotic-resistant bacteria, 7, 43,
    44–45, 83, 97, 99, 113
antibiotics, 7, 20, 21, 29, 30, 35, 36–37,
    47, 81–99, 104, 114, 122, 125,
    202, 224, 231
    allergies to, 92–93, 94
    for chronic infections, 90–91
    decisions about use of, 96–99
    drug interactions and, 92
    follow-up for, 78–79
    function of, 44
    generic vs. brand name, 84–85
    herbal remedies and, 140, 142
    infections not responding to, 107,
        113, 123, 124
    for initial infection, 89–90
    instructions for use of, 43, 45,
        94–96
    intravenous, 91
    overuse of, 82–84
    preventive course of, 90
    recurrent infections and, 42–45, 90
    selection of, 85–93
    side effects of, 93–94
    storage of, 96
    topical, 90–91
    tympanocentesis and, 109–10, 111
    types of, 84–85, 86–89
    waiting to start treatment with, 58
antibodies, 13, 16, 17, 37, 40, 49, 54,
    200, 207
antihistamines, 92, 100, 102–3, 202,
    212–13
antiviral drugs, 36
appetite loss, 19
arnica, 139, 148
aspirin, 101, 125, 137
asthma medications, 92
astragalus, 142, 144
attention deficits, 22
audiologists, 68, 71–75
audiometry, 72–73

auditory evoked responses, 74–75
auditory nerves, 11
    hearing loss and, 23, 24, 74
Augmentin, see amoxicillin clavulanate
azithromycin, 87–88, 92

bacteria, 16, 46, 54
    antibiotic-resistant, 7, 43, 44–45,
        83, 97, 99, 113
    in mouth, inhibiting growth of,
        194
bacterial infections, 16, 17–18, 21,
        32–37, 52
    in AOM, 18–20, 34–35
    in meningitis, 30, 83
    treatment of, 7; see also antibiotics
    vaccinations against, 190–92
Bactrim, see trimethoprim-sul-
    famethoxazole
balance mechanisms, 11
belladonna, 139, 148
Biaxin, see clarithromycin
biologic risk factors, 50–53
bone oscillator, 72, 73–74
books, about going to doctor, 217,
        227–28
bottle propping, 55
brain, 9, 11, 24, 26, 30, 74, 151, 152
breast-feeding, 17, 54–55, 200–201

cancer, 107, 142
caregivers:
    day care, 55–56, 68, 201, 221,
        223–24
    instructions for, 221–23
    medications and, 222, 223–24
cefixime, 87, 90
cefprozil, 86–87, 90
Ceftin, see cefuroxime axetil
ceftriaxone, 87
cefuroxime axetil, 87
Cefzil, see cefprozil
cephalosporins, 83, 86–87, 90, 92
chemotherapy, 107
chiropractic, 8, 133, 136, 150–59
    choosing practitioner for, 172–73
    effectiveness of, 155–56
    precautions for, 158–59
    safety of, 156–57
    in treatment of ear infections,
        157–58
cholesteatoma, 31
chronic serous otitis media, 19, 22–23,
        112, 114, 124, 130, 162–63
chronic suppurative otitis media, 19,
        21, 90–91, 104

cigarette smoke, 54, 68, 199–200
cilia, 40, 52, 54, 103
clarithromycin, 88, 92
cleft palate, 51, 113
cochlea, 11, 24
cold remedies, over-the-counter, 101,
        102, 137
colds, 16, 19, 36, 49, 53–54, 102, 120,
        145, 193, 221
    treatment of, 137, 141, 143, 201–6,
        205
comforting child, 58, 100, 101, 215, 216
complementary and alternative
    medicine (CAM), 7–8, 132–59,
        177, 180, 229–31
    for allergies, 213
    choosing practitioner for, 168–73
    coordination of primary care and,
        176–77
    insurance and, 168–69
    primary doctors and, 135, 143,
        149, 158, 168, 169, 176–77
    scientific evidence on effectiveness
        of, 133–35, 137–38, 145–46,
        155–56
    see also chiropractic; herbal reme-
        dies; homeopathic medicine
conditioned play audiometry, 73
conductive hearing loss, 23–24, 77
corticosteroids, 103–4
Cortisporon Otic, 91
Cotrim, see trimethoprim-sulfamethox-
    azole
cotton swabs, 66, 195–97
coughing, 52, 203, 204
cough remedies, 101, 102
cow's-milk allergies, 211–12
crying, 197
    during doctor's examination,
        63–65, 219
    during hearing tests, 73

day care, 55–56, 68, 201, 221
    medication at, 223–24
decibels (dBs), 75–76
decongestants, 20, 22, 100, 102–3, 197,
        202
dentistry, 194
developmental delays, 25–28
diabetes, 52
diagnosis, 66–68, 178–79, 181
    treatment and, 161–64
diaries, 181, 182
diarrhea, 93
discharge from ear, 19, 21, 58
    after surgery, 109, 118, 119

doctors:
    complementary and alternative
        medicine and, 135, 143, 149,
        158, 168, 169, 176–77
    see also health care providers
doctor's visits, 57–79
    child moving or crying during,
        63–65, 219
    diagnosis in, 66–68
    diagnostic procedures in, 59–63
    discussing treatment options in,
        66–67, 99, 160–64, 179, 181
    follow-up visits, 78–79
    hearing tests in, 67, 68–77
    indicators for, 57–59, 100–101
    preparing child for, 215, 216–19
    rapport with child in, 220
    wax in ear canal and, 65–66
    well-care visits, 25, 184, 217–18
dosages, 94–96, 140
down allergies, 211
Down syndrome, 51–52, 113
dust allergies, 207–8

ear canals, 9, 65
ear drops, 100, 143, 196
eardrums, 9, 12, 13, 18, 19, 24, 66
    assessing function of, 62–63, 70
    differences in, 65
    doctor's examination of, 59–62
    perforation of, 18, 20, 21, 60, 62,
        90, 121, 224
    scarring of, 31, 110, 121
    surgical incisions in, 22, 107–10,
        112, 118, 121
ear infections:
    causes of, 32–49, 164, 181
    children's vulnerability to, 14–17
    complications of, 23–31
    doctor's visits for, 57–79, 100–101,
        215, 216–20
    easing discomfort of, 58, 100, 101,
        215, 216
    health care providers and, 164–82
    inner ear infections, 31, 104
    middle ear infections, see otitis
        media
    outer ear infections, 17–18,
        162–63, 195, 196
    parenting child with, 215–25
    prevention of, 67, 90, 105, 140,
        142, 150, 156, 181, 183–214
    recurrence of, 21, 27, 42–49, 68,
        90, 98, 105, 107, 113, 114, 123,
        162–63, 164
    resolving on their own without

    treatment, 57–58, 105, 114, 133,
        161–64
    risk factors for, 50–56, 68, 98, 107,
        164, 181, 198–201
    symptoms of, 17–23, 57–58
    treatment of, 80–182; see also
        antibiotics; complementary and
        alternative medicine; medica-
        tions; surgery
    use of term, 18
ear pain, 19, 20, 22, 58, 107, 144, 148,
    161
ears:
    anatomy of, 9–13
    healthy, promoting, 194–98
    water in, 195
    wax in, 65–66, 195–97
echinacea, 141, 205
elimination diet, 211
emergency services, 58, 223
ENT (ear, nose, and throat) specialists,
    67, 105, 111, 166, 176, 179
environmental risk factors, 50, 53–56,
    68, 107, 199–200
ephedra, 137, 139
erythromycin-sulfisoxazole, 89, 91
Eryzole, see erythromycin-sulfisoxa-
    zole
essential fatty acids, 41–42
ethnicity, 51
eustachian tube, 18, 21, 34, 36, 40, 41,
    51, 55, 61, 62, 102, 104, 122, 123
    children's vulnerability to ear
        infections and, 14–16
    dysfunctional, 32–33, 54, 113,
        157–58
    functions of, 12–13
    improving function of, 197
    mechanical obstructions of, 32, 33,
        37, 43, 46
    risk factors and, 51, 52

family history, 52
family physicians, 165, 167–68
fats, 41–42, 185
ferrum phosphoricum, 148
fever, 19, 22, 29, 58, 100–101, 107, 144,
    148, 161
flu, 36, 137, 141, 193, 221
fluids, 202, 222
flu shots, 192–93
food allergies, 39, 207, 211–12
Food and Drug Administration, U.S.
    (FDA), 137, 139, 146–47
formula feeding, 54–55, 200–201
frequency, hearing loss and, 77

game-playing, to prepare child for doctor's visit, 217
Gantrisin, see sulfisoxazole acetyl
garlic, 142–43
gender, 51
genetics, 52
ginseng, American, 142, 144
"glue ear," 22
goldenseal, 141, 142, 143
good health, maintaining, 184–87
graperoot, Oregon, 141–42, 143
gum, xylitol, 194

hair cells, 11
head, elevation of, 203
health care providers, 164–75, 231
    alternative medicine practitioners, 168–73, 180
    audiologists, 68, 71–75
    being advocate for your child with, 178–80
    being informed consumer and, 177–78
    choosing, 164–75
    contact information for, 223, 224
    coordinating care between, 176–77, 181
    developing treatment plan with, 66–67, 99, 160–64, 179, 181
    ENT specialists, 67, 105, 111, 166, 176, 179
    general considerations for, 173–75
    partnering with, 8, 160, 180–82, 184
    primary doctors, 164–66, 167–68, 176, 180
    see also doctor's visits
health insurance, 53, 168–69, 179, 223
hearing loss, 21, 22, 23–25, 31, 45, 48, 51, 98, 161, 231
    conductive, 23–24, 77
    developmental delays and, 25–28
    evaluation of, 75–77
    helping child cope with, 225
    monitoring of, 77
    sensorineural (nerve), 23, 24, 74
    signs of, 25
    surgery and, 107, 112, 113, 114
hearing tests, 25, 67, 68–77
    with audiologist, 68, 71–75
    periodic, 77, 79
    preliminary, with doctor, 69–70
    routine screening, 25, 68, 184
Hemophilus influenzae, 30, 34, 35, 43, 89, 90, 190–92
hepar sulph, 148

herbal remedies, 7, 133, 135, 136–44, 177, 213
    for colds, 137, 141, 143, 205
    dosage cautions for, 140
    drug interactions and, 139–40, 143
    effectiveness of, 137–38
    precautions for, 143–44
    safety and risks of, 138–40
    in treatment of ear infections, 140–43
hertz, 77
Hib, 30, 192
histamines, 38
holistic approach, 132
homeopathic medicine, 7–8, 101, 103, 133, 136, 144–46, 169, 177, 206, 213
    choosing practitioner for, 170–72
    effectiveness of, 145–46
    potencies in, 149
    precautions for, 149–50
    safety of, 146–47
    in treatment of ear infections, 147–48
household allergens, 207–11

ibuprofen, 58, 100, 125
immune system, 18, 37, 100, 156
    adenoids and tonsils in, 13, 37, 46
    herbal remedies and, 141, 142
    immature, of infants and young children, 16–17, 51
    nutrition and, 39, 40, 185
immunodeficiencies, 48–49, 52, 53, 54, 164
immunosuppression, 107, 142
immunotherapy, 39, 213–14
infections:
    defense against, see immune system
    protecting your child against, 187–94
    restricting exposure to sources of, 193–94
    see also bacterial infections; ear infections; viral infections
inhaling steam, 204
inner ear, 9, 11, 13
    assessing function of, 73–74
    infections of, 31, 104
insurance, see health insurance
Internet, 177
intravenous antibiotics, 91
intuition, parental, 69
irritability, 19, 20

kali muriacticum, 148, 206

labyrinthitis, 31, 104
laser-assisted myringotomy (LAM), 131
learning problems, 24
lymphatic system, 13, 37, 40, 46, 100

macrolides, 87–88, 92
massage, in chiropractic, 151, 153, 158
mastoiditis, 29, 113
mechanical obstructions, 32, 33, 37,
     43, 46
medical history, 68, 161
medications, 80–104, 181
     for allergic reactions, 212–13
     analgesics, 100–101
     antihistamines and decongestants,
          20, 22, 92, 100, 102–3, 197, 202,
          212–13
     antiviral drugs, 36
     drug interactions and, 92, 139–40,
          143
     generic vs. brand name, 84–85
     instructions for caregiver on, 222
     at school or day care, 223–24
     steroids, 100, 103–4
     see also antibiotics
meningitis, 29, 30, 83
mercurous chloride, 206
middle ear, 9, 11, 40, 102
     assessing function of, 62–63, 66,
          70, 75
     infections of, see otitis media
     ventilation techniques for, 197–98
middle ear fluid, 18–19, 48, 52, 79, 104,
     161
     hearing loss due to, 23–24
     persistent, 45–46, 69
     surgical procedures for, 20,
          106–22, 131
     see also otitis media with effusion
minerals, 40, 185, 186
mold allergies, 199, 208–9, 210
monitoring:
     by caregiver, 222–23
     as treatment option, 80, 97, 98,
          161–64
Moraxella catarrhalis, 35, 43, 89
     vaccination against, 190–91, 192
mouth, 17, 194
mouth breathing, 47, 48, 123, 124
mucus, 36, 38, 52, 54, 120, 203, 204
     drainage of, in eustachian tube, 12,
          16, 40
     removing from nasal passages,
          103, 202–3

myringotomy, 20, 22, 23, 106–11
     benefits and limitations of, 110–11
     follow-up for, 109
     indicators for, 107
     with insertion of tympanostomy
          tubes, 23, 106, 111, 112–22, 123,
          124, 148, 158–59
     laser-assisted, 131
     potential complications of, 110
     procedure for, 108

nasal obstruction, 123, 124
National Institutes of Health (NIH),
     134–35, 138, 155
naturopathic doctors (NDs), 145,
     169–70, 171
neck, 151, 153, 158
nerves, see auditory nerves
nervous system, 151, 152–53
     see also auditory nerve
nonsteroidal anti-inflammatories, 100
nose, 17, 30, 34, 36, 38, 41
nose blowing, 203–4
nose drops, 103, 202–3
nutrition, 185–86
     deficiencies in, 32, 33, 39–42

ofloxacin otic, 91
omega-3 fatty acids, 41
Oregon graperoot, 141–42, 143
ossicles, 11, 24, 30, 31
otitis externa (outer ear infection),
     17–18, 162–63, 195, 196
otitis media (middle ear infections),
     18–23
     chronic suppurative, 19, 21, 90–91,
          104
     complications of, 29–31
     see also acute otitis media; ear
          infections; otitis media with effu-
          sion
otitis media with effusion (OME) or
     middle ear fluid (acute serous
     otitis media), 19, 21–22, 25, 51,
     162–63
     causes of, 33, 35, 37, 38–39, 89, 98,
          163
     chronic, 19, 22–23, 112, 114, 124,
          130, 162–63
     diagnosis of, 61, 66
     follow-up for, 79
     food allergies and, 211
     recurrence of, 27, 42–43, 90, 107
     symptoms of, 22, 162
     treatment of, 35, 81, 98, 100, 102,
          104, 107, 112, 114, 124, 130,

156, 158–59, 163, 197–98
otoacoustic emissions, 72, 73–74
otorrhea, 90, 109, 118, 119
otoscopy, 59–62
    at home, 63, 64
    pneumatic, 61–62
outer ear, 9
    infections of, 17–18, 162–63, 195, 196
overuse of antibiotics, 82–84

pain relievers, 20, 58
parenting child with ear infections, 215–25
    arranging for caregiver or babysitter, 221–23
    comforting child, 58, 100, 101, 215, 216
    easing transition back to school or day care, 223–24
    helping child cope with hearing loss, 225
    keeping child out of school, 220–21
    preparing child for doctor's visit, 215, 216–19
pediatricians, 165, 167
Pediazole, see erythromycin-sulfisoxazole
penicillins, 81–82, 83, 86, 92
pet dander, 209
physical activity, 202, 224
placebo effect, 146
pneumatic otoscopy, 61–62
potassium chloride, 206
preventing ear infections, 67, 90, 105, 181, 183–214
    allergies and, 206–14
    chiropractic and, 150, 156
    cold treatments and, 201–6
    herbal remedies and, 140, 142
    maintaining overall good health and, 184–87
    promoting healthy ears and, 194–98
    restricting exposure to sources of infection and, 193–94
    risk factors and, 198–201
    vaccinations and, 184, 187–93
Prevnar, 30, 191
primary doctors, 164–66, 167–68, 176, 180
    see also health care providers
proving, 147
pulsatilla, 148
pus, 18–19, 29, 58, 90

race, 51
randomized controlled trials, 133–34
reassuring child, 215, 218
recurrences, 21, 27, 42–49, 68, 98, 105, 107, 112–13, 114, 123, 162–63, 164
    antibiotic issues and, 42–45, 90
    chronic adenoid infection and, 46–47
    immunodeficiency and, 48–49
    persistent residual fluid and, 45–46
    reducing risk of, 183–214; see also preventing ear infections
research, 177–78, 181
resources for parents, 227–31
respiratory infections, 18, 19, 34, 40, 46, 49, 52, 53–54, 192, 203
    see also colds; flu
respiratory syncytial virus (RSV), 192
rest, 202, 222
Reye's syndrome, 101
risk factors, 50–56, 68, 98, 164, 181
    biologic, 50–53
    controlling, 198–201
    environmental, 50, 53–56, 68, 199–200
    socioeconomic, 50, 53
Rocephin, see ceftriaxone

saline nose drops, 103, 202–3
school:
    keeping child home from, 220–21
    medication at, 223–24
second opinions, 179–80
semicircular canals, 11, 31
sensorineural hearing loss, 23, 24, 74
Septra, see trimethoprim-sulfamethoxazole
serous (or secretory) otitis media, see otitis media with effusion
sinus infections, 23, 83, 142
skin rashes, 93, 94
sleep disturbances, 19, 20, 123, 124, 130, 215
snoring, 123, 124, 130
social skills, development of, 27
socioeconomic risk factors, 50, 53
sound localization tests, 69–70
specialists, see ENT specialists
speech and language development, 22, 23
    assessment of, 68, 70, 71, 184
    delays in, 25–27, 28, 69, 112, 113
    normal, signs of, 27

speech-language pathologists, 70, 71
spinal column, 151, 152, 153, 154
spinal cord, 30, 152, 153
spleen, 49
*Staphylococcus aureus*, 81
steam inhalation, 204
steroids, 100, 103–4
*Streptococcus pneumoniae*, 30, 34, 35, 43, 83–84, 89, 194
   vaccination against, 30, 189, 190, 191
stress reduction, 187
Sulfatrim, *see* trimethoprim-sul-famethoxazole
sulfisoxazole acetyl, 88, 90
sulfonamides and sulfa combination drugs, 88–89
supplements, 186, 205
suppurative otitis media, 18–21
   chronic, 19, 21, 90–91, 104
   *see also* acute otitis media
Suprax, *see* cefixime
surgery, 7, 24, 29, 77, 98, 105–31
   preparing child for, 116–17
   second opinions and, 179–80
   tonsillectomy, 130–31
   *see also* adenoidectomy; myringot-omy; tympanocentesis; tympa-nostomy tube insertion
swallowing, 12, 22, 124, 197, 198
swimmer's ear, 17–18, 162–63, 195, 196
swimming, 195, 224

tensor veli palatini, 157, 158
throat, 13, 17, 30, 34, 36, 38, 41, 46
thymus gland, 49
tobacco smoke, 54, 68, 199–200
tonsillectomy, 130–31
tonsils, 13, 37
topical antibiotics, 90–91
trans fatty acids, 41–42
treatment, 7–8, 33, 80–164
   developing plan for, 66–67, 99, 160–64, 179, 181
   diagnosis and, 161–64
   evaluating effectiveness of, 77, 78–79
   monitoring and observation as, 80, 97, 98, 161–64
   *see also* antibiotics; complemen-tary and alternative medicine; medications; surgery
trimethroprim-sulfamethoxazole, 88–89
trimethroprim-sulfisoxazole, 91
Trimox, *see* amoxicillin

twenty-four-hour rule, 57–58
tympanocentesis, 106–11
   benefits and limitations of, 111
   follow-up for, 109–10
   indicators for, 107
   potential complications of, 110
   procedure for, 108–9
tympanometry, 62, 66, 70, 75
tympanoplasty, 121
tympanosclerosis, 31
tympanostomy tube insertion, 23, 111, 123, 124, 148, 158–59
   benefits and limitations of, 122
   discussing with your doctor, 113–14
   follow-up for, 118–19
   indicators for, 106, 112–22
   possible complications of, 119–21
   preparing child for, 116–17
   procedure for, 114–18

vaccinations, 30, 35, 36, 83–84, 187–93
   against bacterial infections, 190–92
   standard, 184, 187–90
   against viral infections, 192–93
vancomycin, 83
vertebrae, 151, 153, 157, 158
vertigo, 31, 107
viruses and viral infections, 7, 16, 18–19, 20, 32–38, 43, 46, 54, 201, 221
   antibiotics and, 82, 202
   vaccinations against, 192–93
visual reinforcement audiometry, 73
vitamin C, colds and, 205
vitamins, 185, 186
   deficiencies of, 40–41
voice quality, 67, 70, 71, 130

water in ears, 195
wax in ears, 65–66, 195–97
well-care visits, 25, 184, 217–18
   vaccinations in, 184, 187–93
winter season, 53–54, 193, 201
worry, parent's feelings of, 219
Wymox, *see* amoxicillin

xylitol gum, 194

yawning, 12, 197
yeast infections, 93, 94
yogurt, 93, 94

zinc, 40, 185, 205
Zithromax, *see* azithromycin

# About the Authors

ELLEN M. FRIEDMAN, M.D., received her medical degree from the Albert Einstein College of Medicine in New York and her postdoctoral training in surgery at Montefiore Hospital in New York, in otolaryngology at Washington Hospital Center in Washington D.C., and in pediatric otolaryngology at The Children's Hospital in Boston.

She has had academic appointments in otolaryngology at Harvard Medical School and Boston University School of Medicine and is currently the Dr. Bobby R. Alford Chair of Pediatric Otolaryngology in the Bobby R. Alford Department of Otolaryngology and Pediatrics at Baylor College of Medicine in Houston, Texas. She is also the Chief of Service in the Department of Otolaryngology at Texas Children's Hospital in Houston. In addition to her teaching and clinical responsibilities, Dr. Friedman has conducted research and written numerous articles and chapters on otitis media and related conditions for the lay public as well as for professionals. She is board certified in otolaryngology, is a Fellow of both the American Academy of Pediatrics and the American College of Surgeons, and is a past president of the American Society of Pediatric Otolaryngology.

JAMES P. BARASSI, D.C., received his chiropractic degree from the Palmer College of Chiropractic in Davenport, Iowa, and his postdoctoral training in sports chiropractic at the National College of Chiropractic in Lombard, Illinois. He is currently a Research Fellow in general medicine at Harvard University and Beth Israel Deaconess Medical Center in Boston, and a research consultant in alternative medicine at the Center for Alternative Medicine Research and Education, which is also at Beth Israel.

Dr. Barassi has taught alternative medicine at Harvard Medical School and is currently conducting research in the area of chiropractic for otitis media and for low back pain. He is a diplomate of the American Chiropractic Board of Sport Physicians.